The Osteoporosis Book

The Osteoporosis Book

NANCY E. LANE, M.D.

New York   Oxford
OXFORD UNIVERSITY PRESS
1999

Oxford University Press

Oxford   New York

Athens   Auckland   Bangkok   Bogotá   Buenos Aires
Calcutta   Cape Town   Chennai   Dar es Salaam   Delhi   Florence
Hong Kong   Istanbul   Karachi   Kuala Lumpur   Madrid
Melbourne   Mexico City   Mumbai   Nairobi   Paris   São Paulo
Singapore   Taipei   Tokyo   Toronto   Warsaw

and associated companies in
Berlin   Ibadan

Published by Oxford University Press, Inc.
198 Madison Avenue, New York, New York 10016

Oxford is a registered trademark of Oxford University Press, Inc.

Library of Congress Cataloging-in-Publication Data
Lane, Nancy E.
The osteoporosis book / Nancy E. Lane.
p.   cm.   Includes bibliographical references and index.
ISBN 0-19-511602-X
1. Osteoporosis—Popular works.   I. Title.
RC931.073L366   1998   616.7'16—dc21   98-19650

3 5 7 9 8 6 4

Printed in the United States of America
on acid-free paper

*For my mothers (Sylvia and Betsy),
my role models and mentors;
and for my family and friends,
who have endured*

Contents

Foreword

Osteoporosis is a major public health problem in the United States. Based on data from the Third National Health and Nutrition Examination Survey, which included measurement of bone mineral density at the hip, 20 percent of women and 5 percent of men aged 50 and above in the United States have osteoporosis. Low bone mineral density is the major determinant of increased risk of fracture. An estimated 250,000 hip fractures occur annually in the United States; it is recognized that men and women with hip fractures have high mortality rates, while those who survive the acute hospitalization are at increased risk for long-term disability.

Osteoporosis can be diagnosed easily by measuring bone mineral density at the spine or hip with dual energy x-ray absorptiometry (DXA) or at the forearm or heel with single energy x-ray absorptiometry (SXA) or peripheral-DXA. These techniques are readily available and are covered by Medicare and most insurance companies with the appropriate indication.

Osteoporosis results from a combination of reduced peak bone mass and increased bone loss. Peak bone mass is usually reached in the 20s and depends on hereditary factors during childhood and adolescence. The rate of bone loss during adulthood also depends on calcium intake and exercise, as well as smoking and the occurrence of certain diseases and use of certain medications.

There are now opportunities for both the prevention and treatment of osteoporosis. Prevention of osteoporosis requires an adequate calcium and vitamin D intake, avoidance of smoking, adoption of regular weightbearing exercise, and, in postmenopausal women, use of hormone replacement therapy unless contraindicated for other medical reasons. Numerous medications are now available and approved by the Food and Drug Administration for the prevention and treatment of osteoporosis.

I highly recommend this book for patients with osteoporosis, their family members, and other health-care consumers, as well as health-care providers.

Marc C. Hochberg, M.D., M.P.H.
Professor of Medicine and Head, Division
of Rheumatology and Clinical Immunology,
University of Maryland School of Medicine, Baltimore.
Member, Scientific Advisory Board, National Osteoporosis Foundation.

Why Is This Book Important?

Every day, we look around a busy shopping center and see older women and men who can no longer stand up straight due to a curve in their upper back, or we visit a relative or neighbor in a nursing home who fractured a hip and can no longer live alone. These two scenarios are the result of the disease osteoporosis.

In osteoporosis, the bones become fragile and eventually break. This is a serious health problem because nearly 1 in 4 women over the age of 65, 1 in 2 women over the age of 80, and 1 in 10 men over the age of 80 will get this disease.

Osteoporosis, like many chronic diseases such as heart disease and arthritis, has no early symptoms, and until recently it was not diagnosed until after a fracture had occurred.

Today major advances in our understanding of the life cycle of bone and the treatment of osteoporosis have brought this disease to the spotlight, offering new hope to sufferers and ways to prevent the disease altogether.

This book is about osteoporosis. It discusses the life cycle of bone, who is at risk for osteoporosis, how the disease is diagnosed, and how it is prevented and treated.

The information in this book is critical, allowing every middle-aged woman to be better prepared to prevent osteoporosis. Because the disease is so widespread and, for the most part, is both preventable and treatable, we must start the process of educating ourselves today. Learn about the benefits and risks of estrogen therapy, the other osteoporosis medications that are now available, and the types of calcium supplements that are good for your bones when you are 20 and when you are 75 years of age. Learn about the types of exercise that are good for your bones when you are 40 and when you are 80 years of age.

I wrote this book so that women can understand osteoporosis and how to prevent it, using cases of women and men that most middle-aged women and men can identify with. The methods of preventing and treating this disease are clearly and fully described. It is my hope that with this information the next generation of women and men will all stand tall.

I invite you to read this book and begin the educational process needed to understand the bone life cycle, why we lose bone, and how to prevent this disease.

THE OSTEOPOROSIS BOOK

Introduction

WHY WRITE A BOOK ON OSTEOPOROSIS?

Osteoporosis is a major health problem throughout the world. In people with this disease, the bones become thin and fragile and eventually break. While more women are affected, men suffer as well. This disease threatens 28 million Americans, 80 percent of whom are women. In fact, nearly 40 percent of white women and 13 percent of white men in the United States will have an osteoporotic fracture sometime in their lives. Worldwide, the disease causes nearly 2 million hip fractures each year. Osteoporotic fractures can become life-threatening; nearly 24 percent of elderly people who suffer a hip fracture die within the first year of the fracture, and many others can never live independently again. Osteoporosis, like many chronic diseases such as heart disease and arthritis, has no early symptoms, and until recently it was not diagnosed until after the age of 70 or after a fracture had already occurred.

Recently, major medical advances in the diagnosis, prevention, and treatment of osteoporosis have brought this disease to the spotlight and offered new hope to sufferers. Doctors can now determine, at about age 50 or even earlier, a patient's risk of developing osteoporosis by measuring his or her bone density. Also, several new medications have been approved by the Food and Drug Administration both to prevent osteoporosis and to treat it. And with our growing understanding of the life cycle of bone and of which types of persons risk developing osteoporosis, doctors can now begin to prevent and treat this disease effectively.

This book will describe osteoporosis, who is at risk for developing it, how this disease is diagnosed, and how it is prevented and treated. With this information, you will be better prepared to prevent osteoporosis by taking some necessary precautions. Because this disease is so widespread, we must start the process of educating ourselves today.

WHAT IS OSTEOPOROSIS?

People with osteoporosis have fragile bones because their bone mass is low and the structure of the bone is poor. The combination of low bone mass and changes in bone structure leads to bone fragility, and many people with osteoporosis will suffer fractures. This definition of osteoporosis emphasizes *bone or skeletal fragility*—the key concept that links low bone mass (a condition called *osteopenia*) with a risk of fractures, the consequence of osteoporosis. In fact, if it were not for fractures, osteoporosis would not be such an urgent medical problem. Fractures can occur in the spine, hip, wrist, ankle, pelvis, and ribs. In fact, almost all bone fractures that occur in postmenopausal women and elderly men are osteoporotic fractures because the bone has become thin and weak. With very little trauma, the bone breaks.

Until recently, osteoporosis could only be diagnosed after a patient experienced a fracture. But now, with the use of bone density measurements, bone mass can be assessed before a fracture occurs. We will discuss how bone density is measured and how osteoporosis is diagnosed.

We have all recognized women with osteoporosis whose spinal vertebrae have fractured. They look hunched over and may also have a "dowager's hump," or *dorsal kyphosis*, in their upper back. Often these women notice that they have lost several inches in height since they were young adults.

But osteoporosis does not happen all at once; it usually develops over several decades, influenced by how much bone mass we have in early adulthood. We build bone mass until about the age of 20 to 30 and then maintain it until about the age of 50 in women and 70 in men. After the age of 50, women lose bone during menopause from estrogen deficiency and later due to age-related factors including changes in calcium balance, inactivity, and other illnesses. After about the age of 60, once bone mass has declined over a period of 10 years, bone mass becomes so low that a cough or a fall can bring on a cascade of events that may be irreversible. With one fall and one hip fracture, the individual may never regain independence and may decline through inactivity and fear of falling again. Unfortunately, doctors see these patients only after they have already suffered a fracture and a decline. I have written this book so that both women and men can take steps to prevent this disease.

WHO GETS OSTEOPOROSIS?

Among white women living to 80 years of age, about one-third will have one hip fracture and many will have two. Overall, a white woman who lives to this age has nearly a 50 percent chance of having an osteoporotic fracture of the spine, the hip, or the forearm. Men also get osteoporosis, but they do not tend to lose much bone until after the age of 70, so fractures do not occur until they are well into their 80s. However, nearly 13 percent of white men will have an osteoporotic fracture in their lifetime. Because so many people are affected, the risk factors for this disease will be discussed in detail.

TOPICS IN THIS BOOK

The structure and life cycle of bone and how osteoporosis develops are covered in Chapter 1. Persons who have a risk of developing this disease will be identified in Chapters 2 and 4. Osteoporosis in men is covered in Chapter 5; diagnosis is discussed in Chapter 3. Strategies that can be used to prevent the disease are described in Chapters 6 to 9, and treatment of existing osteoporosis is presented in Chapters 8 to 12.

Part I
UNDERSTANDING OSTEOPOROSIS

1

Understanding the Life Cycle of Bone

WHAT IS BONE TISSUE MADE OF?

There are two types of bone tissue. *Cortical bone* makes up 80 percent. It is solid and dense, giving the skeleton most of its strength. The other 20 percent is *trabecular bone*, which is made up of a fine lattice network that surrounds the bone marrow. Although this lattice network is very thin, it provides maximum support with a minimum amount of material. All of these fine surfaces create an enormous amount of exposed area, and because of its closeness to the bone marrow, rapid changes in bone mass can occur in the trabecular bone. For this reason, bones that have a large percentage of trabecular bone, such as the spine, are susceptible to disturbances in the bone life cycle.

Each bone consists of both types of bone tissue, with trabecular bone inside, next to the bone marrow, and cortical bone surrounding it. The amounts of cortical and trabecular bone differ from one bone to another and even within the same bone. The vertebrae of the spine are composed mostly of trabecular bone surrounded by a thin cortical shell. At the other extreme, the long bones of the arms and legs are mostly made up of cortical bone, with trabecular bone concentrated only at the ends of the bones.

Bone tissue is composed of tiny crystals of calcium and phosphorus embedded in a framework of interlocking protein fibers. The main protein in the bone is collagen type 1. The calcium crystals give the bone strength, hardness, and rigidity; the collagen fibers provide flexibility. Other minerals are also present in bone, including fluoride, sodium, potassium, citrate, and other trace minerals. These other minerals function as glue, holding the calcium and phosphorus crystals together.

HOW DO WE GAIN AND LOSE BONE THROUGHOUT LIFE?

To understand osteoporosis, you must understand bone. To begin with, remember that our bodies are very efficient machines. Bone maintains its tissues by a carefully planned maintenance cycle. In fact, almost all body tissues are constantly being maintained or replaced throughout life, and bone tissue is no exception. Bone tissue is constantly replaced, or *turned over*, by removal of old tissue and replacement with new tissue. This process is known as the *bone remodeling cycle*, and we will look at it in some detail. Bone remodeling occurs when small amounts of bone are lost or broken down by cells known as *osteoclasts*. After this small amount of bone is lost, or *resorbed*, a *resorption pit* is formed on the bone. Another type of cell, or *osteoblast*, moves into the area of bone that has been lost and replaces it with new bone. This process continues on small parts of all of our bones throughout life. Bone mass is maintained by the delicate balance of these two processes (Figure 1.1). The bone remodeling cycle can change in response to different needs of your body. The entire cycle can take 4 to 8 months but can range from as little as 3 months to as long as 2 years. Resorption is rapid, taking only 4 to 6 weeks; new bone formation is slow, taking up to 2 months for each remodeling cycle.

HOW DOES AGE AFFECT YOUR BONES?

All parts of the body change as we age, and the skeleton is no exception. From the time of birth until you reach adulthood, or about 30 years, you make more bone tissue than you lose. But after 30, the reverse is true: you lose more bone than your body makes.

Bone has three surfaces, or *envelopes*, and each envelope has different anatomical features, even though its cell makeup is identical to that of the other two. The bone surface facing the marrow cavity is known as the *endosteal envelope*, the outer surface is the *periosteal envelope*, and the bone in between is the *intracortical envelope* (Figure 1.2). In childhood, new bone is formed on the periosteal envelope and a smaller amount of breakdown occurs on the endosteal envelope. Children grow because the amount of bone formed in the periosteum exceeds what is broken down on the endosteal surface of the cortical bone.

During adolescence, growth is accelerated due to increased sex hormone production. Estrogen and progesterone in girls and androgen (testosterone) in boys stimulate the formation of new bone on the periosteal surface of the cortical envelope. Later in adolescence, more bone is added to the inner surface and in the *intracortical envelope*. The growth spurt that occurs in adolescence is due to the laying down

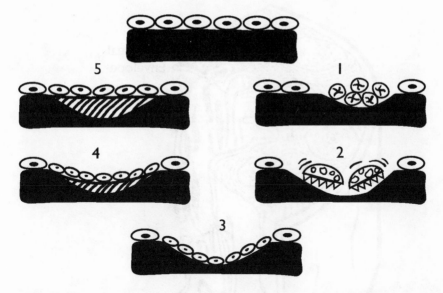

Figure 1.1 *The bone remodeling cycle. Bone remodeling consists of a series of steps, and the normal bone remodeling cycle takes about 4 to 8 months. The stages of this cycle are as follows: (1) Osteoclasts are recruited to the bone surface; (2) osteoclasts erode the bone surface, dissolving the bone mineral and matrix and producing a resorption cavity; (3) osteoblasts are attracted to the resorption pit; (4) osteoblasts form new bone and fill the resorption pit; and (5) the bone surface is covered with lining cells.*

of new bone tissue on both the inner and outer surfaces of existing bone. This pattern of bone growth continues until about the age of 20 to 25, with the pattern of bone remodeling consisting of outer surface formation and inner surface breakdown. In later adulthood, the rate of breakdown exceeds the rate of formation and bone mass begins to decline.

IS THE BONE LIFE CYCLE DIFFERENT IN WOMEN AND MEN?

Both women and men lose bone as they grow older; the difference is in the amount of bone loss and the rate of loss. Bone mass begins to decline in both sexes in the early 30s, with very small losses of trabecular bone from the spine (Figure 1.3). Women lose bone much more rapidly than men; by the age of 80, a woman may have lost over 40 percent of her trabecular bone mass, while a man may have lost only 13 percent. Cortical bone mass reaches its peak at around

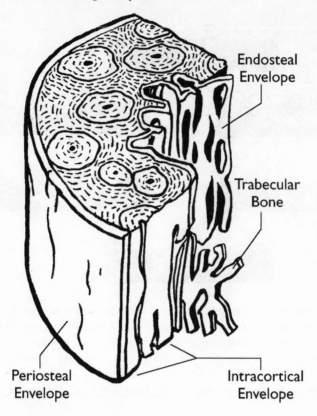

Figure 1.2 *The three surfaces, or envelopes, of bone and trabecular bone.*

age 20 to 25; from then until about the age of 50, both sexes experience a slight loss, usually from the long bones of the arms and legs.

Women also lose bone rapidly in the first 7 to 10 years following menopause because of a decrease in estrogen. The amount of bone that each women loses during menopause varies, as we will discuss in the next chapter. The rate of bone loss during menopause is six times faster than that of a man, and a new pattern of bone remodeling occurs at menopause, exactly the opposite of the growth pattern of adolescence. If a woman does nothing to prevent the bone lost at menopause, by the age of 55 to 57, or 5 years after menopause, the amount of bone she gained during adolescence (her estrogen-dependent amount of bone) will have been lost.

At about the age of 60 to 65 years, the rate of bone loss in women begins to slow down and becomes similar to that of men. But it is important to remember that even though the rate of bone loss slows, a woman may have already lost as much as 20 percent of her bone

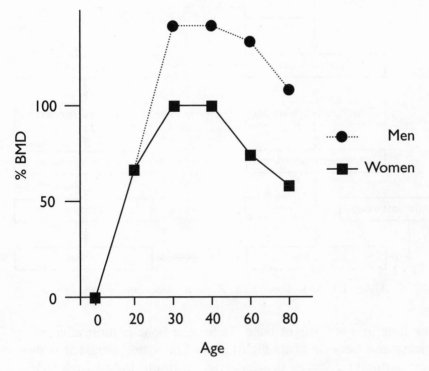

Figure 1.3 *The changes in bone mass density (BMD) with age.*

mass. Men and women will continue to lose bone as they age, about 1 or 2 percent a year; this slow, steady bone loss is a natural part of the aging process. Although we generally think that the bone loss of aging is slow and continuous, we are now finding that when activity changes, or when we become immobilized or ill with another disease, bone loss accelerates. The reasons for accelerated bone loss with be covered in other chapters.

WHAT HAPPENS IN MENOPAUSE?

As a woman enters menopause ovarian function declines, reducing production of two hormones, estrogen and progesterone. A woman knows that she has entered menopause when her menstrual cycle ends. As the estrogen (estradiol and estrone are the estrogens in the bloodstream) levels fall, the bone remodeling cycle changes and loss of bone tissue begins. One function of estrogen is to maintain the normal rate of bone remodeling. When the estrogen levels falls in menopause, bone resorption becomes greater than bone formation,

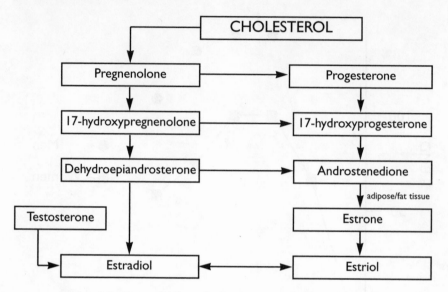

Figure 1.4 *The metabolic pathways for the production of estrogen.*

resulting in a net loss of bone. Trabecular bone is most affected by menopause because of its high turnover rate and because it is most susceptible to estrogen deficiency. As a result, trabecular bone becomes thin and eventually perforated or disconnected from its surrounding tissue. Over time, when enough bone has been disconnected, the trabecular bone weakens. The loss of these trabecular connections is one of the reasons that bone becomes weak and eventually breaks or fractures.

While many menopausal women respond to estrogen deficiency with an increase in their bone remodeling cycle and loss of a significant amount of bone, some women do not. In menopause, the ovaries produce less estrogen and progesterone, but the ovary is not the only source of estrogen (Figure 1.4). Fat, or adipose, tissue produces androstenedione, which is converted into estrogen. In general, women who weigh more and have a higher fat content tend to lose less bone in menopause. In fact, researchers measuring the changes in bone mass after menopause are finding that the rate of bone loss varies widely. Some women lose as much as 5 percent of their bone mass a year for 3 to 5 years, while others lose much less; the reasons for this variability are not completely understood.

The bone loss that results in osteoporosis and painful fractures is present for a long time in the asymptomatic, or silent, phase. The analogy that is often used to understand the links between bone mass and osteoporosis is the relationship between high blood pressure, a silent symptom, and the dramatic onset of heart disease. The disease processes that change bone mass or increase blood pressure have no symptoms. It is only when a patient has a heart attack or an osteoporotic fracture that the problem comes to the attention of the doctor and the patient. Thankfully, regular medical checkups allow patients to have their blood pressure monitored so that hypertension can be treated and heart disease prevented. And now, with bone densitometry, the risk of osteoporosis can also be detected and treatment begun, if necessary, to prevent disease. Menopause is the time when bone loss usually begins, and it is then that a woman's risk of osteoporosis can be detected and prevented.

The impact of osteoporosis in women after menopause is dramatic. Seventy-five percent of the vertebral fractures and 50 percent of the hip fractures they suffer are believed to be the result of bone loss that accompanies or begins at menopause.

WHAT HAPPENS AS WE AGE? TYPE I AND TYPE II OSTEOPOROSIS

We have been focusing on osteoporosis resulting from bone loss during menopause in women, but fractures are also due to bone loss with aging. Bone loss from estrogen deficiency that results in osteoporosis is often referred to as *postmenopausal* or *type I osteoporosis*. Another type of osteoporosis, *age-related* or *type II osteoporosis*, occurs with aging and affects both men and women after the age of 70.

In age-related bone loss, there is an "uncoupling" or imbalance of the bone remodeling cycle. As we age, calcium absorption becomes more difficult. Vitamin D helps us absorb calcium, but with age it does not seem to work as well. When this occurs, less calcium is available. The body reacts by producing more parathyroid hormone, which pulls calcium from the bone through resorption. If this occurs, bone resorption increases and less bone is replaced.

Aging, in general, slows the rate of bone formation for each bone's remodeling cycle. As a result, more bone is resorbed than is formed; thus, over time, more bone is lost than made. Fortunately, this type of bone loss is slow. The resulting fractures affect both the cortical and trabecular bones—primarily those of the hip and spine, upper arm, ribs, and pelvis. The previously mentioned dowager's hump, or dorsal kyphosis, reveals the dramatic bone loss that may occur in the spine (Figure 1.5).

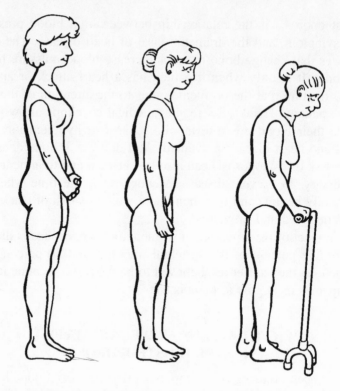

Figure 1.5 *A dowager's hump, or dorsal kyphosis.*

MEDICAL CONDITIONS THAT CAN CAUSE OSTEOPOROSIS

Many medical conditions can accelerate bone loss and result in fractures of the hip and spine. These include cancers, especially multiple myeloma (cancer of plasma cells made in the bone marrow), hyperthyroidism (overactive thyroid gland), early menopause or surgical removal of the ovaries (oopherectomy), hypogonadism (low testosterone level) in men, stomach surgery with partial removal of the stomach (subtotal gastrectomy), paralysis of one side of the body from a stroke or neurological disease (hemiplegia), Cushing's syndrome (a pituitary gland tumor that creates overproduction of glucocorticoid hormones that regulate glucose metabolism, and glucocorticoid excess results in bone loss), and systemic mastocytosis (a disease of white cells). These conditions all affect bone mass in different ways. Multiple myeloma results in overproduction of plasma cells in the bone marrow, causing loss of bone mass. In hyperthyroidism, the overproduction of thyroid hormone results in high bone resorption. Testosterone is the hormone the maintains bone mass in men, just as estrogen does in women. Thus, a low testosterone level in men results in bone loss. Stomach surgery can cause bone loss because calcium absorption is reduced. Paralysis on one side of the body results in inactivity and thus in bone loss. Finally, in Cushing's syndrome, the excess glucocorticoids produced by the tumor can cause bone loss (see Chapter 11).

HOW DOES THE BODY MAINTAIN ITS CALCIUM LEVEL?

Ninety-five percent of your body's calcium is present in your bones. However, calcium is critical not only for healthy bones but also for every system and process in the body, including muscle contraction, blood clotting, brain function, heart rhythm, and kidney function. Because calcium is so important, the body has developed an elaborate system of hormones to keep the calcium level constant in the blood. The most important of these substances are parathyroid hormone, vitamin D, and calcitonin.

Parathyroid hormone is made in the four tiny parathyroid glands tucked in behind the neck and attached to the thyroid gland. Parathyroid hormone controls the calcium level in the blood. If this level falls below a certain point, this hormone is released into the bloodstream and increases the calcium level in the blood in a number of ways. Since calcium is critical to brain and cell health, bone mass may be sacrificed to ensure that an adequate level of calcium is maintained in the bloodstream.

Vitamin D is obtained primarily from the sun, where it is produced by the ultraviolet irradiation of an inactive form of the vitamin in the skin. It is also found in small amounts in eggs, milk, and fish. Vitamin D is stored in the liver in a partially activated form and is transported to the kidney, where it is converted into its final, active form. Once activated, vitamin D increases the absorption of calcium from the intestines and stimulates the kidney to reabsorb calcium from the urine back into the bloodstream. Vitamin D, like parathyroid hormone, is responsible for maintaining a specified level of calcium in the blood. So, the correct amount of vitamin D is important to maintain calcium balance.

Several substances can affect vitamin D levels in the body. Anticonvulsant drugs stimulate the production of liver enzymes that break down vitamin D, which can lead to a vitamin deficiency. Patients on anticonvulsants can develop osteomalacia from the vitamin D deficiency and osteoporosis from the resulting calcium deficiency. This bone loss can be avoided if the doctor regularly monitors the calcium and vitamin D levels in these patients.

Calcitonin, another hormone, is made in the thyroid gland. It appears to protect bone from the resorption effects of parathyroid hormone. As we will discuss in later chapters, calcitonin is used for treatment of osteoporosis.

SUMMARY

- Bone tissue is constantly replaced (turned over) in the bone remodeling cycle, a lifelong process.
- We all gain bone mass until about the age of 20 to 25 years.
- From age 30 to age 50 in women (30 to 70 in men) bone mass remains stable until women go through menopause.
- Beginning at menopause, women lose bone rapidly as their estrogen level drops. This loss of bone mass remains a silent problem until a fracture occurs.
- Both men and women develop age-related bone loss in their 70s due to the calcium imbalance of aging, sedentary lifestyle, and other conditions.
- Calcium, an important mineral for bone health, helps bone grow strong in youth, maintains bone mass in middle age, and prevents some bone loss with aging. Vitamin D increases calcium absorption.

2
Who Is At Risk of Developing Osteoporosis?

WHAT IS BONE MASS?

Many studies show that low bone mass leads to osteoporosis. But what is bone mass, and how is it measured?

A single bone mass measurement at any commonly assessed site (forearm, heel, finger, hip, or lumbar spine) predicts the overall risk of fractures in women. Bone mass measurements also predict the risk of specific types of osteoporotic fractures, including those of the wrist, upper arm, hip, and most other sites. The site of a bone mass measurement can be important. For example, bone mass measured at the hip is a better predictor of hip fracture than bone mass measured at other sites. The relationship of bone mass to fractures is quite strong. For example, if a woman's hip bone mass is 20 percent below normal for her age, she is about seven times more likely to have a hip fracture than a woman whose hip bone mass is 20 percent above normal for her age. The lower the bone mineral density, the higher the risk of having a fracture. In chapter 3, we will see that the definition of *low bone mass* or *fracture threshold* is arbitrary, though it may be useful when deciding which therapy to use.

Bone mass in an elderly woman reflects a combination of the woman's peak bone mass at about 30 years of age and the subsequent rate of loss. Rates of bone loss at menopause can vary considerably, not only between individuals but also in the same individual at different stages of life. Therefore, there is no age at which it is too late to prevent fractures by preventing bone loss.

AGE, SEX, AND RACE

Age, sex, and race are among the strongest determinants of bone mass and fracture risk. In general, African-Americans have the highest bone mass, while whites, particularly those of Northern European descent, have the lowest. The bone mass of Asian-Americans is somewhere in between. We do not know all the reasons that African-American women have more bone mass, but we do know that these women have larger bones at skeletal maturity. Studies show that even at an early age, there are differences between African-American and white children. African-American women usually have a higher muscle mass. Bone mass and muscle mass are closely related in that the bigger the muscles, the higher the stress on the bones and the larger the bones. Also, aging African-American women appear to lose bone less rapidly than their white counterparts. This may be due to hormonal differences between the two races. What this may mean is that if you are an African-American woman, you will probably have greater bone mass when your skeleton matures, so that more bone must be lost before you develop osteoporosis. This is not true of all African-American women; some do experience osteoporotic hip fractures, but they tend to be older than white women when these fractures occur. Also, an African-American woman whose ovaries are removed at an early age and who is not treated with hormone replacement therapy has the same risk of developing an osteoporotic fracture as a white woman whose ovaries were removed at a young age, although the African-American woman will have some protection because she probably started with a higher bone mass.

Few studies have focused on other ethnic groups. In general, women with ancestors from Northern European countries, Japan, and China are more likely to develop osteoporosis than those of African, Hispanic, or Mediterranean ancestry. The risk for women of Middle Eastern ancestry seems to lie between those of African-Americans and whites. Perhaps skin pigmentation and the distance one lives from the equator are related to the overall risk of osteoporosis; for example, white women who have a fair complexion and live far from the equator, in countries like Sweden or Norway, have a high risk of osteoporosis. In a dark-complexioned African woman, on the other hand, the risk of osteoporosis is quite low.

FAMILY HISTORY AND REPRODUCTIVE FACTORS

Genetic factors do contribute to our bone mass and can predispose us to or protect us from osteoporosis. Studies of twins suggest that peak bone mass in the hip and spine is largely determined by genetic factors, and there may even be a genetic component to the rate of bone loss. Daughters of women who have had an osteoporotic fracture have, on average, slightly lower than normal bone mass for their age (3 to 7 percent lower, on average). A family history of an osteoporotic fracture is useful in assessing a person's risk of fracture.

Estrogen deficiency at the time of menopause is linked with accelerated bone loss in women. When estrogen levels fall after menopause, bone is resorbed more vigorously. However, the rate of bone loss and the risk of fracture vary greatly among women entering menopause.

Removal of the ovaries before natural menopause greatly increases bone loss and the risk of hip fractures. A woman who has had a shorter reproductive span because of late menstruation (after the age of 15) or early menopause will have low bone mass, and this effect persists into old age. Several reproductive factors, including having very few pregnancies, a short breast-feeding history, and menstrual irregularities may be associated with low bone mass or fractures in postmenopausal women, but these relationships are not clear.

BODY TYPE

Low body weight, low body mass index (a measurement of weight divided by height), and decreased muscle strength are all associated with decreased bone mass in both sexes in all areas of the body. Some studies suggest that the effects of weight on bone mass are greater at weight-bearing sites—for example, the upper leg or femur, or the lower leg or tibia. In women, weight may influence bone mass primarily through its effect on the skeleton. Women who weigh more put more stress on their bones, and since increased stress stimulates new bone formation to meet this higher demand, bone mass can increase.

Obese women rarely develop osteoporosis. Although the reasons are not completely understood, obese and slender women differ in their ability to produce estrogens after menopause. Before menopause, the ovaries produce large amounts of estrogen and progesterone and small amounts of other male hormones, such as androgens. The adrenal glands also produce androgens. After menopause, very small quantities of estrogen and progesterone are produced, but the same amounts of androgens are produced as before menopause.

In fat, or adipose, tissue, androgens can be converted into estrogen. The more fat tissue a woman has, the more estrogen she can produce. Fat, therefore, greatly reduces a woman's risk of developing osteoporosis. Also, soft tissue padding may protect the skeleton from trauma and fractures. But while some fat may prevent osteoporosis, there are important reasons not to gain too much weight. An obese woman has a higher risk of developing cancer of the uterus, an estrogen-dependent cancer. This may happen because she is producing estrogen in her fat but her ovaries are no longer producing progesterone, which normally protects against uterine cancer. Therefore, the estrogen-progesterone imbalance can predispose a woman to cancer after menopause. Increased fat mass is also associated with an increased risk of breast cancer and heart disease. Therefore, we need to eat a balanced diet and to remember the risks and benefits of weight gain when it comes to healthy aging.

Weight loss in the elderly person as compared to the young adult is also associated with low bone mass, while weight gain is associated with high bone mass. Why weight loss in the elderly affects bone mass is not entirely clear. Most likely, the lower stress of reduced body mass, the lower level of estrogen, and other illnesses all play a role. Also, weight loss can result in weakness of the arms and legs, which can increase the risk of falling and fracturing.

BIRTH CONTROL PILLS

Birth control pills have been used for over 30 years. Most of us have heard about the bad effects of some of these medications; few have learned about their benefits. There is some evidence that women who have used birth control pills for a long time have stronger bones than those who have not. Oral contraceptives contain a combination of estrogen and progesterone, both of which may increase bone mass. It has been suggested that the extra amounts of these hormones protect these women from loss of bone mass and may even stimulate some bone formation. More research is needed to determine the protective effects of birth control pills. In Chapter 9, we will look at how oral contraceptives protect some young women athletes against the risk of stress fractures.

LIFESTYLE FACTORS

Lifestyle behaviors such as smoking cigarettes, drinking alcohol, and being physically active affect the health of all of us, both directly and indirectly. We are just beginning to sort out these complicated relationships.

Smoking

Tobacco smoke may be toxic to bone. It may also increase the liver's breakdown of estrogen, so that estrogen levels are lower in smokers than in nonsmokers. Postmenopausal women who smoke and take estrogen still have significant bone loss. Smokers also weigh less and can have an earlier menopause (about 5 years earlier) than nonsmokers, all of which could account for their higher risk of osteoporosis. Smokers are one and a half to two and a half times more likely to have hip and wrist fractures (women) and vertebral fractures (women and men).

Alcohol Use

Heavy use of alcohol for many years results in reduced bone mass, greater bone loss in postmenopausal women, and more fractures. Alcohol may have a directly toxic effect on bone tissue or it may affect bone mass through poor nutrition because heavy drinkers usually do not eat a healthy diet and derive most of their calories from alcohol. Also, liver disease from heavy alcohol use may alter the way vitamin D is metabolized, which may, in turn, impair calcium absorption and result in weakened or abnormal bone. Heavy drinking may also increase the risk of falls that result in fractures. In fact, it can result in osteoporosis in both men and women as early as their 30s. The influence of moderate alcohol use, about one to two drinks a day, on bone mass and fractures is not clear.

Physical Activity

Weight-bearing exercise stresses the skeleton and causes muscle contractions that stimulate bone formation. Conversely, prolonged immobility or inactivity from bed rest leads to bone loss. A lifetime of vigorous physical activity leads to slightly higher bone mass, and athletes generally have somewhat greater bone mass than nonathletes. Exercise regimens that are vigorous and emphasize muscle strength training preserve and may even increase bone mass in adults and may prevent falls. And there is no age limit to the benefits of exercise on bone mass, muscle strength, and balance. However, we are uncertain about the ability of moderate exercise, such as walking, to prevent bone loss. In Chapter 9, we will discuss exercise and its role in preventing osteoporosis.

Even though strenuous exercise has only a modest effect on bone mass, several studies have found that elderly women and men who exercise regularly generally have a lower risk of hip fracture. This finding is consistent with research on osteoporosis resulting from immobility and a sedentary lifestyle. Elderly women who are on their feet less than 5 hours a day have nearly twice the risk of hip fracture of more active women. Therefore, even small amounts of weight-bearing activity may have important benefits in old age.

Calcium and Vitamin D Intake

Calcium is a major component of bone, so it is logical to assume that a low-calcium diet means unhealthy bones. While we often state that osteoporosis in women is the result of estrogen deficiency, it is equally true that it is a problem of calcium deficiency.

As people age, their ability to absorb calcium from the gastrointestinal tract declines; by the age of 80, most women absorb less than half of the calcium in their diets. This is probably one of the reasons we lose bone as we age. The reduced calcium absorption is increased by low calcium intake. Also, as they age, both men and women develop some deficiency in lactase, the enzyme necessary to digest milk, causing them to eat less calcium-rich foods. Finally, at menopause, calcium absorption is reduced due to estrogen deficiency—another reason that women lose more bone than men.

In the early 1980s, researchers found that a high proportion of older American women took in less than 500 milligrams of calcium a day. This finding was dramatic because the recommended daily allowance (RDA) of calcium is 1200 to 1500 milligrams for a postmenopausal woman. Therefore, a high percentage of elderly American women ingest only a third of the calcium that they need each day. (Chapter 7 covers the calcium requirements for bone health at all ages.) Low calcium intake results in bone loss because it stimulates the release of parathyroid hormone, which pulls calcium out of the bone. The longer a woman has a low calcium intake, the weaker her bones will be.

Whatever the amount of calcium you currently take in supplements and food, if you are menopausal and not taking estrogen replacement therapy, you will absorb less calcium and excrete more of it than someone who is premenopausal or someone who is menopausal and receiving therapy. Thus, women need more calcium after menopause than before.

The amount of calcium required to maintain or protect your bone mass after menopause increases from an RDA of 800 to 1000–1200 to 1500 milligrams. If you are a typical American woman over the age of 45, you consume far too little calcium because foods high in calcium are also high in calories; you also may have a problem digesting these foods. The average calcium intake of American women over the age of 45 is about 450 milligrams a day. These women are depleting their bone mass by about 1.5 percent per year. At this rate, a woman who goes through menopause at the age of 50 will have lost 15 percent of her bone mass by the time she is 60 and 30 percent of her bone mass by the time she is 70, from calcium loss alone. The good news is that that population studies show a small but consistent increase in bone mass in women with higher daily calcium intakes (including diet and supplements),

Men, like women, have a problem absorbing calcium as they age. The major cause of age-related bone loss in men is altered calcium balance. At around the age of 75, men require about 1200 milligrams a day of calcium to maintain a normal calcium balance. Elderly men require calcium supplementation just like elderly women.

The role of calcium deficiency in osteoporosis must be considered together with vitamin D deficiency. Severe vitamin D deficiency causes *osteomalacia*, a failure to mineralize bone tissue. Housebound, institutionalized, and elderly persons who live in very cold winter climates have a high risk of developing severe forms of vitamin D deficiency. Bone loss due to vitamin D deficiency may be at least partially prevented by taking vitamin supplements. A study of nursing home residents in their mid-80s found that a calcium supplement of 500 milligrams a day plus 800 international units (IU) of vitamin D per day—the amount found in two multivitamin tablets—reduced the risk of hip fractures and other nonspine fractures by about one-third over an 18-month treatment period. Therefore, for elderly men and women who are especially prone to calcium and vitamin D deficiency, these supplements can prevent bone loss and reduce fractures.

Diet

Protein
Childhood malnutrition, which affects protein intake, and prolonged vitamin D deficiency have significant effects on skeletal development and the peak bone mass of young women. Although we do not know

if malnutrition results in an increased risk of fractures, it seems likely because poor diet usually delays puberty, and delayed puberty is a clear risk factor for osteoporosis.

Young women also can suffer from anorexia nervosa, a disease that usually occurs in those who do not eat because they are concerned that food will make them appear heavy and unattractive. Anorexia may be so severe that the young woman will literally starve to death. Although we know that anorexia can lead to low bone mass in young women, we do not yet know if malnutrition results in an increased risk of fracturing. However, a low peak bone mass in an adult does increase a woman's lifetime risk of fractures.

A high-protein diet may increase the risk of osteoporosis. When animal protein is broken down in the body, it produces acid. This acid is buffered in the bone by releasing calcium, which is lost in the urine. We do not yet know how high the protein content of a diet must be to result in bone loss or to increase the risk of fractures.

To confuse matters, while we know that protein is important for strong bones, it is also true that a vegetarian diet may protect against bone loss. A study compared older white women who ate meat regularly to lacto-ovo-vegetarians who ate only cheese and diary products; the vegetarians had lost far less bone with age. Both the meat eaters and the vegetarians had good amounts of calcium in their diets, yet the meat eaters lost about a third of their bone mass between the ages of 50 and 90, while the vegetarians lost only a fourth. Another study of both men and women showed that vegetarians had more bone mass in their 70s than had meat eaters in their 50s. The reasons for this difference in bone loss are not completely clear. Red meat is high in phosphorus and may change the phosphorus-to-calcium ratio, resulting in calcium loss. Another explanation may be the acid levels of the two diets. A vegetarian diet is low in acid, while a meat diet is high. This acid must be neutralized, and this occurs in the bone. To move the acid from the bloodstream to the bone, calcium must be moved out of the bone. This movement of the acid into bone and calcium out of bone causes a net loss of calcium from bone. Over time, this calcium loss may result in lost bone mass and fractures. However, a balanced diet with 45 grams of protein daily does not cause calcium loss if the ratio is maintained—i.e., 45 grams of protein plus 1000 milligrams of calcium.

Phosphorus

Phosphorus is an essential mineral found in every cell in your body, and it is involved in almost every metabolic process. Along with calcium, phosphorus is a major component of bone. But some scientists believe that if the phosphorus in your diet exceeds the calcium, bone loss can occur. Many foods, such as bread, cereal, potatoes, red meat, and cola-containing drinks, contain much more phosphorus than calcium. Also, phosphorus is widely used in food additives and is a major component of processed foods.

We don't yet understand exactly how this imbalance of phosphorus and calcium results in bone loss. It is possible that a diet high in phosphorus may increase parathyroid hormone (which moves calcium out of the bone) and cause calcium to be lost from the urine. It is probably safe to say that a teenager whose diet is high in phosphorus compared to calcium may lose calcium in the urine, and over time this may reduce one's ability to achieve peak bone mass.

Caffeine

Some researchers have found that people who consume a lot of caffeine have an increased risk of osteoporosis, but not all of them agree. A high caffeine intake means six or more cups of coffee or tea a day. Moderate intake of caffeine probably does not increase the risk of low bone mass and fractures as long as enough calcium is also obtained. If caffeinated beverages are substituted for calcium, then the calcium deficiency may be the cause of bone loss, not the caffeine. A recent study of elderly women found that high intake of caffeine resulted in low bone mass for their age, but if they had a sufficient amount or the RDA of calcium, their bone mass was normal. For now, it appears that high caffeine intake may be a risk factor for low bone mass, especially if the caffeinated beverages replace calcium in the diet.

DRUGS THAT CAUSE OSTEOPOROSIS

There are medications that, if taken for a long time, alter bone turnover and increase the risk of osteoporosis. These include steroids, thyroid hormone of thyroxine, gonadotropin-releasing hormone (GNRH) analogs (used to treat endometriosis or uterine fibroids and prostate cancer), anticonvulsants (antiseizure medications) like Dilantin®, diuretics like Lasix®, and anticoagulants (blood-thinning medications) like heparin. At this time, steroids and thyroid medications are the most common drugs that lead to drug-related osteoporosis. We will review these medications briefly here.

Thyroid Medications

Thyroid medications, including Synthroid® and thyroid extract (or L-thyroxine), are prescribed for many people who have too little thyroid hormone. The thyroid gland produces thyroid hormone, which controls the metabolic rate of the body. If the thyroid gland is underfunctioning or the person is *hypothyroid* (has too little thyroid hormone), he or she will feel tired and may gain weight. On the other hand, if the person feels very energetic, and perhaps has a slight hand tremor and weight loss, the thyroid gland is overfunctioning and the person has too much thyroid hormone, or *hyperthyroidism*. When too much thyroid hormone is produced, bone turnover is also faster, resulting in more bone resorption than formation and a net loss of bone. People who are hypothyroid are treated with thyroid medications.

For a long time, thyroid hormone extract was derived from the cow's thyroid gland and used to treat hypothyroid patients. It was difficult to standardize the dose. Many patients were given too much thyroid hormone and lost bone, experiencing all the symptoms of osteoporosis, including fractures. Physicians monitored the circulating thyroid hormone either with a radioimmunoassay (a test that tagged the circulating thyroid hormone with a radioactive tag that allowed it to be counted) or with other tests that were not as standardized as they are now. Today a physician monitors thyroid hormone replacement by measuring the thyroid-stimulating hormone (TSH) level. When the thyroid hormone level in the circulation is normal, the TSH is in the normal range. When a hypothyroid patient is given too much thyroid hormone, the TSH level is below normal. Several studies show that in this situation, an individual has low bone mass and may have an increased risk of developing an osteoporotic fracture.

Thus, hyperthyroidism can increase bone turnover and, over time, cause bone loss, with an increased risk of osteoporosis. Too much thyroid hormone replacement used for the treatment of hypothyroidism can increase bone loss and put the person at risk of developing osteoporosis. Individuals who have been hyperthyroid and those who have been on thyroid hormone replacement therapy should have their bone mass measured. Too much thyroid hormone, either produced naturally or given as medication, can result in a few years in bone loss and increase an individual's risk of developing osteoporosis.

Steroids

Another common cause of drug-induced osteoporosis is steroid-induced bone loss. Steroids are used to treat several inflammatory, noninfectious diseases, including such chronic diseases as asthma, rheumatoid arthritis, inflammatory bowel disease, multiple sclerosis, and skin diseases like chronic dermatitis. Steroids are potent anti-inflammatory drugs. In high doses they are also immunosuppressive, that is, they decrease the function of the the immune system. They are the best medications we now have to reverse acute inflammatory reactions like anaphylaxis (severe allergic reactions), skin reactions to poison oak, and severe asthma attacks. Many patients need to take steroids on a regular basis to keep their disease under control. People who have severe rheumatoid arthritis, systemic lupus erythematosus, or even severe asthma must take a low but regular dose of steroids to manage their disease. But while steroids help to keep diseases under control and are lifesaving, they have many other effects on the body, especially on bone.

Steroid-induced bone loss is a very complex process. Steroids directly prevent osteoblasts from maturing and making new bone, resulting in bone loss during each remodeling cycle. Steroids also prevent calcium absorption and increase calcium loss. These changes in calcium metabolism can cause an increase in parathyroid hormone and thus an increase in bone resorption to maintain the calcium balance. Finally, steroids decrease the production of the sex hormones, called *gonadal hormones*—estrogen in women and testosterone in men—resulting in further bone loss.

The dose of steroids that can cause bone loss is low. Prednisone, for example, at 7.5 milligrams a day, or its equivalent of another steroid, can cause bone loss. At a dose of 7.5 milligrams a day for 6–12 months, prednisone results in a loss of 10 to 20 percent of spinal trabecular bone. After the initial rapid loss of trabecular bone, steroids cause a slow but continual loss of both cortical and trabecular bone of 1 to 2 percent per year. Both men and women of all races taking steroids appear to lose bone mass. The bone loss can be even greater if the patient is not very active because steroids can cause loss of muscle mass, or muscle wasting. Prolonged use of steroids leads to muscle wasting, and less muscle mass means that there is less muscle pull or stress on the bone, so more bone is lost. This time the loss is from the cortical bone. Individuals taking steroids may also be weak and inactive due to their primary disease, such as asthma or rheumatoid arthritis. These people will probably remain inactive and thus tend to have greater bone loss on steroids.

It was once believed that every-other-day steroid therapy did not result in steroid-induced bone loss, but this is not true. Although bone loss may be slowed on this schedule, prolonged use still results in significant bone loss. Moreover, people who take inhaled steroids for the treatment of respiratory diseases can also develop steroid-induced bone loss if they inhale over 1000 micrograms of steroid a day (a dozen sprays a day).

Steroid-induced osteoporosis is diagnosed the same way as postmenopausal osteoporosis. One difference, however, is that steroid-induced osteoporosis appears to result in rib fractures rather than the more common hip fractures seen in postmenopausal women.

Now that we understand the process of steroid-induced bone loss, we can effectively prevent or treat it, a topic that we will take up in Chapter 11.

GNRH Agonists

Gonadotropin-releasing hormone (GNRH) agonists are medications that increase the release of this leutinizing hormone and follicle-stimulating hormone from the pituitary gland. These hormones (LH and FSH), once released, move through the bloodstream to the ovary or the testes, where they stimulate the release of estrogen or testosterone. At first, GNRH agonists increase LH and FSH production, but then very quickly, within 7 to 10 days, the production of these hormones significantly decreases; after 14 days of this treatment, estrogen or testosterone falls to below-normal levels. These drugs are used to treat women who have endometriosis or fibroid tumors in the uterus. In men, they are used to treat prostate cancer. Women usually take these medications for 6 months; during the treatment period, lumbar spine bone mass decreases by 7 to 10 percent. Although these women tend to be young or premenopausal, if they have several treatment periods with these medications, they will have substantial bone loss and an increased risk of osteoporosis. When these drugs are prescribed, it is critical to discuss prevention of bone loss with your physician.

Men are given GNRH agonists to treat prostate tumors. Although we know less about the resulting bone loss in men, GNRH agonists do lower testosterone levels, and testosterone, like estrogen in women, maintains bone mass in men. When testosterone levels fall to around 50 percent of normal, bone loss occurs. It is important for men taking these drugs to discuss how to prevent bone loss with their physician.

Diuretics

Diuretics such as furosemide (Lasix®) and hydrochlorothiazide promote urine production and are often prescribed for people who have high blood pressure or heart disease. In terms of their effects on bone mass, some diuretics are good and others are bad. Furosemide increases urinary calcium excretion; if there is no increase in calcium intake, bone loss can result. On the other hand, thiazides decrease calcium excretion. Studies have found that elderly women who take thiazide diuretics for many years have a higher bone mass and fewer osteoporotic fractures than women of the same age who do not take these medications. However, although thiazides may prevent bone loss, a woman must take them for over 10 years to achieve this effect.

Antacids

Women constitute an increasing number of the over 3 million Americans who have ulcers. These women, plus a greater number of women who do not have ulcer disease, are daily users of antacids.

Most people consider these medications to be harmless and do not realize that they may contain aluminum, which can increase calcium loss in the urine; if this occurs, calcium will be pulled from the bones to keep the calcium level normal in the bloodstream. Aluminum-containing antacids themselves do not usually cause osteoporosis, but they are often used together with steroids to decrease the gastrointestinal symptoms that often occur with those medications. Alcoholics often take antacids on a regular basis to soothe their stomachs, and this combination can be very destructive to bone mass. Not all antacids are harmful to bone mass, but neither men nor women should take aluminum-containing antacids unless they are prescribed by a physician.

SUMMARY

- Low bone mass leads to osteoporosis.
- Many factors determine bone mass: age, sex, race, and genetics are the most important; weight, medications, and lifestyle factors are others. The combination of the bone mass you inherit, your lifestyle, and your diet affect your risk of developing osteoporosis. Some determinants of low bone mass are reversible; others are not.
- Low body weight, low body mass index, and decreased muscle strength are linked to decreased bone mass in both men and women.
- Long-term use of birth control pills may strengthen bones somewhat.
- Smoking may be toxic to bone, promotes estrogen breakdown, and leads to weight loss and early menopause.
- Long-term heavy alcohol use reduces bone mass and increases bone loss after menopause. Heavy drinkers have a poor diet and do not absorb vitamin D well, which may impair calcium absorption.
- A sedentary lifestyle leads to loss of bone. Vigorous exercise preserves bone mass, and regular exercise reduces the risk of hip fracture.
- A high-calcium diet is important throughout life. Supplements (at least 1000 milligrams per day until menopause, 1500 milligrams per day thereafter) are also important.
- The best diet is moderately high in protein, with plenty of fruits and vegetables.
- Drugs that lead to osteoporosis include steroids, GNRH analogs, thyroid drugs, diuretics, and antacids with aluminum.

3
How Do We Diagnose Osteoporosis?

HOW CAN I TELL IF I HAVE OSTEOPOROSIS?

The question every woman needs to ask is, am I at risk of developing osteoporosis? How can I know if I have already lost bone mass? No one should wait until a painful vertebral fracture occurs to find out that they are losing bone. The key questions are: How much bone do I have now? How rapidly am I losing it?

HOW IS OSTEOPOROSIS DETECTED?

Until very recently, detection of osteoporosis was difficult. Usually by the time this condition was apparent to a doctor or a patient, extensive and irreversible bone loss had already occurred. For example, about 40 percent of a woman's bone mass must be lost from the thoracic or lumbar spine before it can be seen with a regular X-ray. But if 40 percent of a woman's bone mass is gone, the woman is already osteoporotic and has a very high chance of fracturing. Women sometimes notice that they have lost a few inches in height and/or that they have developed a hump in their upper back. These women have already sustained vertebral compression fractures; they now have irreversible bone loss and osteoporosis.

Like other chronic diseases, such as atherosclerosis or high blood pressure, osteoporosis is silent; there are no signs or symptoms before a fracture occurs. But we have developed accurate, precise ways to measure bone mass so that a woman can know her risk of developing osteoporosis. The advances in osteoporosis detection are similar to those in heart disease, in which a measurement of cholesterol can assess a person's risk of developing atherosclerotic vascular disease. Although neither a cholesterol measurement nor a bone mass measurement alone can completely define a person's risk of developing these diseases, they are very helpful.

WHAT ARE THE SIGNS AND SYMPTOMS?

The diagnosis of osteoporosis can be made by finding a fracture of the vertebrae, of the hip, of the wrist, or of any other bone in an older woman or man. But how do we detect osteoporosis if there have been no fractures?

In women both with and without fractures, measurement of bone mass can tell us her current bone mass and risk of future fractures. Bone mass measured at any part of the skeleton also can assess the risk of a woman's having a fracture. Over the past 10 years, several noninvasive techniques have become available to measure bone mass. Let's look at some of them.

TECHNIQUES FOR MEASURING BONE MASS

Many techniques have been used to assess bone mass. These methods determine the bone mineral content of the whole skeleton, the forearm or heel, or the lumbar spine or hip. We measure bone mass because it is correlated with bone strength. This means that the more bone mass you have, the higher the load required to induce a fracture. The best predictor of a future osteoporotic fracture is bone mass. Therefore, a bone mass measurement is a very important diagnostic tool.

Conventional Radiographs or X-rays

Conventional X-rays, like a back X-ray, cannot detect bone loss. Usually, as mentioned earlier, about 40 percent of bone mass must be lost before it can be seen on an X-ray. However, X-rays are valuable for determining the presence of osteoporotic fractures that have already occurred unknown to the patient.

Single Photon Absorptiometry

Single photon absorptiometry (SPA) was the first truly automated methods used to measure bone mass. A densitometer measures the mineral content of the bones of the forearm by calculating how many gamma rays are absorbed; the greater the absorption, the greater the bone mineral content and the greater the bone density.

The procedure is simple. The scanner is aligned with the forearm and measures the bone density at the distal forearm. The instrument is connected to a computer that calculates the results and prints them out in graph form. The results show the actual bone mineral density in your forearm and the percentage of bone that you have compared to people of the same age (Z score) and compared to young, healthy adult bone mass (T score). The test is painless, takes less than 10 minutes, and exposes you to less than 1/100th the amount of radiation in a normal X-ray.

SPA measures both types of bone, cortical and trabecular. In the forearm, especially the lower end of the radius, about 26 percent of the bone is trabecular. Therefore, an SPA measurement of bone mass at that location involves a high percentage of trabecular bone. A measurement at the middle of the forearm involves about 70 percent cortical bone.

SPA offers a simple, noninvasive measure of bone skeleton status and has good precision and accuracy. Over the past 5 years, most SPAs have been replaced by single X-ray absorptiometers (SXA). The SXA is just as accurate as the SPA, but instead of using an isotope and counting gamma rays, it uses an X-ray source; the amount of radiation is small, and the X-ray source does not lose strength over time.

Dual-Energy X-ray Absorptiometry

Bone sites such as the spine and the hip are surrounded by various amounts of soft tissues, including fat, muscle, blood vessels, and abdominal organs. These tissues limit the use of SPA or SXA because they cannot penetrate through the soft tissues; they can only be used for bones that are close to the skin. Dual-energy X-ray absorptiometry (DXA) allows us to measure the mass of both superficial and deeper bones.

The lumbar spine is measured with the patient lying on her back (Figure 3.1). The legs are either flat or elevated to reduce the curve at the lower back and to make the back as straight as possible. The spine scan lasts about 5 to 10 minutes. The computer generates a report of the bone mineral content, the bone mineral density, and the percentage of bone mass for the subject's age (Z score), as well as a comparison to a young, healthy adult (T score).

The hip or the proximal femur is another commonly measured site for a DXA scan. Bone mass can be measured for the total hip or the individual parts of the hip, including the femoral neck, the trochanter, the intertrochanteric region, and Ward's triangle (Figure 3.2). The

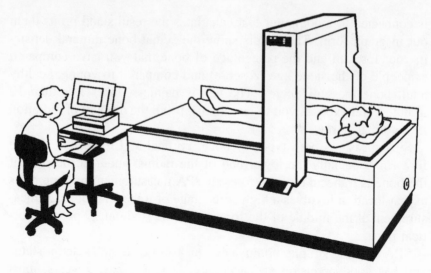

Figure 3.1 *The bone mineral density of a patient's spine is measured by DXA.*

whole region of the femur or hip area is scanned, and sites of interest are selected with computer assistance.

The DXA scanner can also be used to measure total body bone mineral content and bone mineral density at the distal forearm and heel.

The radiation exposure from the DXA scans is very low, probably about 1/100th that of a normal X-ray. This makes them safe for both initial and repeat bone mineral density scans if necessary.

Quantitative Computed Tomography

The best way to determine early trabecular bone loss in the spine is with a specially modified quantitative computed tomography (QCT) scanner. The procedure takes about 20 minutes. The patient lies on her back, while the measurement is taken at the midportion of the first and second lumbar vertebrae in the lower back. The measurement is important because it can give an accurate measurement that is 100 percent trabecular bone mass, with no cortical bone (the outer envelope of bone) or other artifacts. This measurement can be used to calculate a woman's risk of a vertebral fracture. It is important to remember that a bone fractures because of loss of both cortical and trabecular bone, and DXA can easily obtain this measurement. This technique, however, is generally used only for research purposes because of the high cost of purchasing the instrument and running the

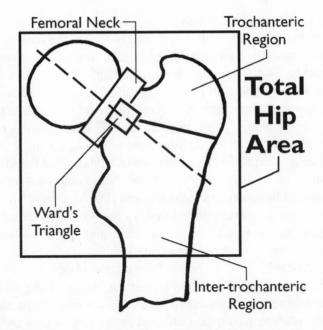

Figure 3.2 *The different regions of the hip measured in a bone mineral density scan by DXA.*

QCT. In addition, the radiation required to perform a good QCT scan for trabecular bone is much higher than that required for DXA, SPA, and SXA. For these reasons, it is not generally used to measure or monitor bone mineral density.

Peripheral Quantitative Computed Tomography

Recently, a peripheral QCT (PQCT) scanner has been developed that can measure forearm trabecular bone and both cortical and trabecular bone. The radiation dose is about the same as that of a regular X-ray of the arm. Although the radiation dose is lower than that of the QCT used to measure spinal BMD, it is still much higher than that of the other bone measurement techniques available. At this time, this technique can be used to assess the risk of osteoporotic fractures in the peripheral skeleton.

Ultrasound Measurement of Bone

Ultrasound techniques are used to diagnose many disorders. In diagnosing osteoporosis, a quantitative ultrasound (QUS) device measures the speed of a sound wave traveling through bone. If the bone is thick, the sound wave will travel slowly. But if the outside cortical bone is thin and the interior trabecular bone is sparse, the sound will travel quickly. Therefore, the transit time of the ultrasound wave may be related to the amount of bone and to the trabecular structure in the bone's interior. Researchers are trying to determine whether the ultrasound measurement gives an indication of bone quality, or structure, that is superior to the information provided by the usual bone mass techniques. Most of the studies seem to show that the ultrasound measurement gives different information about bone mass but is equal to the standard bone density measurement (DXA) in predicting future fractures. Since the bone mineral density measurement tells us something about the amount of bone we have and the ultrasound measurement tells us something about the quality of the bone, together they can probably give us better information about an individual's risk of developing an osteoporotic fracture. Some of the early QUS bone measurement instruments required that the bone being measured be placed in a water bath or stabilized in some sort of stand. Moreover, these early instruments could only measure bones that were very close to the skin, such as the kneecap or the heel. The new versions being tested allow the ultrasound probe to be placed on the outside of the lower limb (the tibia), and good information has been obtained this way.

The bone mass measurement techniques discussed above are summarized in Table 3.1.

All bone mineral density techniques have relatively low radiation exposure (similar to that of a standard chest X-ray). QUS uses only sound waves and has no radiation at all.

What Does the Bone Mineral Density Test Tell Us?

Over the years, several groups of researchers have developed techniques to diagnose osteoporosis on the basis of bone mass measurements. At this time, the most conventional method defines a *fracture threshold*, a cutoff point for bone mineral density at which most patients will have a very high risk of developing an osteoporotic fracture. The cutoff point depends on several factors, including the bone that is measured, the site of interest, and the patient's age and sex.

In adult women, the cutoff value of 2.5 standard deviations below

Table 3.1. *Bone Mass Measurement Techniques*

Technique	Name	Sites Scanned	Scanning Time (minutes)
SPA	Single photon absorptiometry	Radius Calcaneus (heel)	5–10
DXA	Dual-energy X-ray absorptiometry	Lumbar spine	5–10
		Lateral lumbar spine	15–20
		Femur (or hip)	5–10
		Total body	20
QCT	Quantitative computed tomography	Lumbar spine	20
		Femur	20
PQCT	Peripheral quantitative computed tomography	Forearm	10
QUS	Quantitative ultrasound	Kneecap	15–20
		Lower leg	10–15
		Heel	10–15

the average bone mass for a young, healthy adult, or a T score of less than −2.5, is a reasonable cutoff point for most patients who have a hip fracture. The standard deviation refers to a normal distribution of bone mass in a population of 30-year-old women; 1.0 standard deviation below the normal bone mass, or a T score of −1, means that a subject's bone mass is 10 percent less than the normal value. A T score of −2.0 indicates bone mass 20 percent less than the normal peak bone mass value, and a T score of −2.5 shows bone mass about 25 percent below the peak bone mass. This cutoff point permits four general diagnostic categories for bone mass to be established for adult women. These categories have been accepted by the National Osteoporosis Foundation of the United States, the World Health Organization (WHO), and the European Foundation for Osteoporosis and Bone Diseases. These four diagnostic categories are as follows:

1. *Normal.* A value for bone mineral density or bone mineral content not more than 1 standard deviation below average for young adults, or about 10 percent below the young adult average or higher.
2. *Low bone mass (osteopenia).* A value for bone mineral density or bone mineral content more than 1 standard deviation below the young adult average, but not more than 2.5 standard deviations below the young adult average or 10 to 25 percent below this average.
3. *Osteoporosis.* A value for bone mineral density or bone mineral

content more than 2.5 standard deviations below the young adult average value, or 25 percent below this average or less.

4. *Severe osteoporosis (established osteoporosis).* A value for bone mineral density or bone mineral content more than 2.5 standard deviations below the young adult average value, or 25 percent or more below this average and the presence of one of more osteoporotic fractures.

According to these guidelines, about 30 percent of postmenopausal women have osteoporosis using bone mineral density measurements made at the spine, hip, or forearm.

Osteoporosis increases exponentially after the age of 50 in women, and so does the incidence of osteoporotic fractures. The number of women with low bone density increases with age, making the number of elderly women at risk for an osteoporotic fracture significantly higher. Although we know that low bone density, or a T score of −2.5 at the hip, means that a woman has a high risk of developing a hip fracture, we cannot be certain that she will have a fracture. This concept of disease differs from that of other diseases; for example, with breast cancer, an individual either has or does not have the disease, even though it may exist at one of various stages.

A bone mineral density measurement is similar to a cholesterol blood test that gives an individual a defined risk of developing heart disease (see the three cases at the end of this chapter). With osteoporosis, low bone density is the risk factor, and you visit the doctor when you have a fracture, a clinical sign of the disease. With coronary artery disease, high cholesterol is the major risk factor, and the clinical sign of the disease is a heart attack. Therefore, a certain cholesterol level assigns an individual a certain risk for developing coronary artery disease. In the same way, a bone mineral density measurement assigns an individual a certain risk of developing an osteoporotic fracture. And depending on your bone mineral density measurement, there are specific treatments and guidelines applicable to you.

HOW DO WE MEASURE BONE LOSS AND GAIN OVER TIME?

Once you have received a diagnosis of osteoporosis or low bone mass, your doctor will want to continue to monitor bone loss or gain over time. Measurements of bone loss or gain are obviously important for the diagnosis and management of osteoporosis. The most direct way to measure changes in bone mass is to perform another bone mass measurement. Bone measurement devices have improved over the past 5 years and can now be used to reliably measure changes in bone mass. Currently, there are no solid recommendations on when a women should have another bone mass measurement. Generally, if a woman starts to use a medication that affects her bone mass, like estrogen, a repeat bone mass measurement can be done 1 year later. Modern bone mass measurement devices have about a 1 to 2 percent margin of error. Keeping this in mind, and depending on the patient's expected bone loss, the doctor will decide whether to remeasure the woman's bone density in 1 or 2 years or later. An example is the use of a bisphosphonate to treat osteoporosis. This treatment is expected to increase bone mass by 2 to 3 percent per year. In this case, a repeated bone mass measurement after 1 to 2 years can determine if a woman is responding to the treatment.

CAN BLOOD TESTS DIAGNOSE OSTEOPOROSIS?

A lot of research is being done to find markers in the blood and urine that can give us information about the activity of bone cells and to determine whether the markers can indicate bone loss, bone gain, or a response to therapy.

Unlike bone mass measurements, which assess the bones themselves, biochemical markers provide information about the activity of the disease in the body. Changes in bone turnover and bone loss can be detected in several of the body's activities: calcium metabolism, collagen turnover, bone protein turnover, and the activity of bone cells themselves.

Calcium Measurements in Blood (Serum) and Urine

In postmenopausal osteoporosis, serum (the liquid part of blood) calcium and phosphorus levels are usually normal, and measurements of these elements in the urine are also relatively normal. In osteoporosis, calcium loss from the bone is increased but calcium loss from the urine remains relatively normal. In all forms of osteoporosis there is increased calcium loss from the bone. This can sometimes cause a small increase in serum or blood calcium, but it is somewhat offset by a decrease in calcium absorption, so that the calcium loss in urine over 24 hours is generally in the normal range. If calcium in the urine does become high, this may be due to increased gastrointestinal absorption or another event that dramatically increases bone resorption—such as prolonged bed rest, which greatly increases the amount of calcium released into the bloodstream and then excreted in the urine. Measurements of calcium in the urine can be used to assess the patient's response to therapy. For example, a treatment that decreases bone resorption also decreases calcium excretion, and a treatment that increases bone formation also may decrease calcium excretion.

Alkaline Phosphatase

Alkaline phosphatase, an enzyme, is frequently used as a blood marker for skeletal disease because it is a product of the osteoblast cells, (the cells that form new bone). In adults, about half of the alkaline phosphatase is derived from the bone and the other half comes from the liver. A test has been developed to measure alkaline phosphatase activity in bone, and this test is becoming increasingly popular. In osteoporosis, bone-specific alkaline phosphatase activity is usually increased. In early menopause, bone turnover (both formation and resorption) increases about twofold and may remain elevated for several years, then start to decrease.

Collagen Breakdown

Collagen is the major protein present in bone and skin. When collagen breaks down, hydroxyproline, a major body protein, is excreted. When bone turnover increases, so does the excretion of hydroxyproline. Hydroxyproline values increase about twofold or more after menopause.

Several laboratory tests have been developed to measure a small part of the collagen protein in the bone, called *collagen cross-links*. When the collagen in the bone is broken down by the osteoclast cells that resorb bone, collagen cross-links are released from the bone and excreted essentially unchanged. These small cross-links have been found to correlate with the bone resorption activity of the osteoclasts. When bone resorption goes up, the level of the collagen cross-links excreted into the urine increases. Physicians can use these tests to monitor bone cell activity and the patient's response to therapy.

Osteocalcin

Osteocalcin is a protein made by the osteoblasts, the bone-forming cells. While it is not part of the bone tissue itself, it is released into the bloodstream and therefore can be used to measure bone formation. Since bone turnover, including bone resorption and formation, increases early in menopause and probably never returns to premenopausal levels, osteocalcin levels increase at menopause and remain higher than before menopause for the rest of a woman's life.

Biochemical markers that signal bone turnover are used by your doctor to assess disease activity and to estimate the rate of bone loss. A measurement of bone mass does not tell you whether bone is currently being lost or gained. This measurement assesses your risk of developing an osteoporotic fracture. Meanwhile, measures of bone cell activity, or turnover, provide information about the rate of bone loss. The latter measures also give information about the effects of a treatment so that in the near future they may make repeated bone mass measurements unnecessary.

Studies suggest that the rate of bone loss in women in early menopause can be accurately predicted by the use of biochemical markers. The higher the bone turnover, as indicated by these markers—that is, the higher the level of bone resorption compared to bone formation—the higher the rate of bone loss. Ongoing studies are focusing on how much information the biochemical markers can tell us about the rate of bone loss and what an individual's future risk of fracture will be. These markers of bone turnover will probably provide very useful information to both patients and doctors about the rate of bone loss, the response to therapy, and the future risk of fractures.

BONE MINERAL DENSITY SCAN OF THE LUMBAR SPINE WITH THE CLINICAL INTERPRETATION

Figure 3.3 is a DXA scan of the lumbar spine of a 53-year-old woman who underwent a total hysterectomy (uterus removed) and a bilateral ovariectomy (both ovaries removed) at the age of 40. The scan shows the four lumbar vertebrae identified and measured. The bone mineral content (BMC) values are shown for each vertebral level. For these values, the bone mineral density (BMD) of each vertebra and of the four lumbar vertebrae together (L1–L4) is computed. For this woman, the BMD is 0.736 grams per centimeter squared (gms/cm^2). In the graph next to the scan, the BMD is plotted against a reference graph for the age and sex of the patient. The middle line in the graph is the normal BMD for each age for a woman. The upper and lower lines represent two standard deviations above and below the BMD for each age. The dotted line represents the lower level of BMD for young, healthy premenopausal women. The patient's lumbar spine BMD is

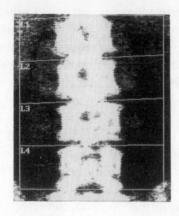
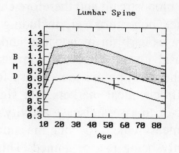

Region	Area (cm2)	BMC (grams)	BMD (gms/cm2)
L1	14.14	9.27	0.656
L2	15.32	11.21	0.732
L3	16.44	12.73	0.774
L4	17.01	13.06	0.768
TOTAL	62.90	46.27	0.736

Region	BMD	T(30.0)		Z	
L1	0.656	-2.45	71%	-1.61	79%
L2	0.732	-2.69	71%	-1.76	79%
L3	0.774	-2.82	71%	-1.83	79%
L4	0.768	-3.16	69%	-2.15	76%
L1-L4	0.736	-2.83	70%	-1.87	78%

* Age and sex matched
T = peak bone mass
Z = age matched

Figure 3.3 *Bone mineral density scan of the lumbar spine with the clinical interpretation.*

below this level; it is −2.83 standard deviations below average (T score). The Z score represents the number of standard deviations below that expected for her age and sex. In this case, the BMD of L1–L4 results in a Z score of −1.87—that is, almost two standard deviations below the BMD expected for the patient's age and sex. The cause of this woman's low spinal BMD is no doubt the removal of her ovaries 13 years ago, resulting in premature or surgical menopause, and failure to provide treatment to prevent bone loss. She has osteoporosis (T score below −2.5) and has a very high risk of having an osteoporotic fracture in the near future. This patient is definitely a candidate for treatment.

BONE MINERAL DENSITY SCAN OF THE HIP WITH THE CLINICAL INTERPRETATION

Figure 3.4 is a DXA scan of the hip of a 59-year-old woman who has been postmenopausal since the age of 51. She has not been taking any medications to prevent bone loss, eats a normal diet, and has no medical problems. The BMC values are shown for each area of the

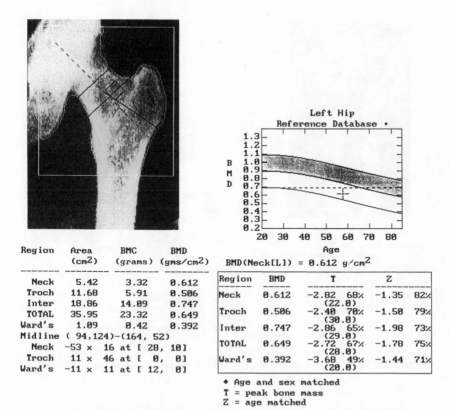

Region	Area (cm2)	BMC (grams)	BMD (gms/cm2)
Neck	5.42	3.32	0.612
Troch	11.68	5.91	0.506
Inter	18.86	14.09	0.747
TOTAL	35.95	23.32	0.649
Ward's	1.09	0.42	0.392
Midline	(94,124)-(164, 52)		
Neck	-53 x	16 at [28, 10]	
Troch	11 x	46 at [0, 0]	
Ward's	-11 x	11 at [12, 0]	

BMD(Neck[L]) = 0.612 g/cm²

Region	BMD	T		Z	
Neck	0.612	-2.82	68%	-1.35	82%
		(22.0)			
Troch	0.506	-2.40	70%	-1.50	79%
		(30.0)			
Inter	0.747	-2.86	65%	-1.98	73%
		(29.0)			
TOTAL	0.649	-2.72	67%	-1.78	75%
		(28.0)			
Ward's	0.392	-3.68	49%	-1.44	71%
		(28.0)			

♦ Age and sex matched
T = peak bone mass
Z = age matched

Figure 3.4 *Bone mineral density scan of the hip with the clinical interpretation.*

hip that has been scanned. For these BMC values, the BMD of each area and of the total hip bone is computed. For this woman, the BMD for the total hip is 0.0.649 g/cm². In the graph next to the scan, the BMD is plotted against a reference graph for the age and sex of the patient. The middle line in the graph is the normal BMD from 20 to 80 years of age. The upper and lower lines represent two standard deviations above and below the BMD for each age. The dotted line represents the lower level of BMD for young, healthy premenopausal women. The patient's BMD is below that level; her total hip BMD is −2.72 standard deviations below average (T score). The Z score represents the number of standard deviations below that expected for her age and sex. In this case, the BMD of the total hip results in a Z score of −1.78, which is also low. This woman has very low bone mass, and her risk of developing an osteoporotic fracture is high. Reasons for her very low bone mass may include 9 years of estrogen

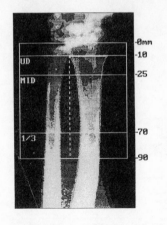

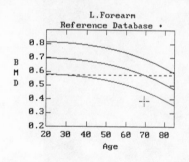

RADIUS	Area (cm2)	BMC (grams)	BMD (gms/cm2)
UD	3.57	0.93	0.260
MID	7.11	2.34	0.329
1/3	3.12	1.20	0.384
TOTAL	13.80	4.46	0.323

BMD(Radius[L] 1/3) = 0.384 g/cm^2

Region	BMD	T		Z	
1/3	0.384	-5.17 (20.0)	55%	-3.15	67%
MID	0.329	-5.08 (20.0)	54%	-3.07	66%
UD	0.260	-3.15 (20.0)	59%	-1.71	72%
TOTAL	0.323	-4.73 (20.0)	56%	-2.80	68%

♦ Age and sex matched
T = peak bone mass
Z = age matched

Figure 3.5 *Bone mineral density scan of the forearm with the clinical interpretation.*

deficiency and a possible family history of osteoporosis of which she may be unaware. She should begin therapy immediately.

BONE MINERAL DENSITY SCAN OF THE FOREARM WITH THE CLINICAL INTERPRETATION

Figure 3.5 is a DXA scan of the left forearm of a 70-year-old woman who has been postmenopausal since the age of 50. She started estrogen replacement therapy when she went through menopause, but she stopped the treatment within a year and has taken no estrogen replacement therapy for the past 19 years. The BMC values are shown for each area of the forearm that was measured. The BMD measurement of the forearm is divided into four sections. The ultradistal radius (UD) is the part of the bone area just next to the wrist. The mid region of the radius (MID) is the part of the forearm farther away from the wrist. The 1/3 distal radius area is located approximately in the middle of the radius bone and is an area rich in cortical bone. The total forearm BMD measurement represents the BMD measurement for the other three areas. For the BMC values, the BMD of each area and of the total area is computed. For this woman, the ultradistal BMD is 0.93 g/cm². In the graph next to the scan, the BMD is plotted against a reference graph for the age and sex of the patient. The middle line in the graph is the normal BMD for each age listed below for a woman. The upper and lower lines represent two standard deviations above and below the BMD for each age. The dotted line represents the lower level of BMD for young, healthy premenopausal women. This patient's BMD is far below this level; the 1/3 radius BMD is 5.17 deviations below the average of the young adult (T score). The Z score represents the number of standard deviations below that expected for the patient's age and sex. In this case, the BMD of the 1/3 radius is −3.15—that is, over three standard deviations below normal for her age. This woman may not have achieved a normal peak bone mass in young adulthood, and since she has not been taking estrogen replacement therapy for the past 19 years, preventable further bone loss has occurred.

SUMMARY

- Osteoporosis, or low bone mass, is detected by a bone mass measurement (bone densitometry) using many different methods. Today, bone densitometers can easily measure bone mass at the forearm/wrist, spine, hip, or total body bone mass and give the exact bone mass of a man or woman. It can also indicate how this bone mass compares to that of normal persons of the same age and sex (Z score) and how it compares to the peak bone mass (T score).
- Bone mass density measurements tell us our risk of developing an osteoporotic fracture.
- Blood tests are available to show how actively bone is remodeling; however, they cannot show what degree of osteoporosis exists.

4

Bone Fractures and Osteoporosis

RISK FACTORS IN ELDERLY PERSONS

Most nonspine fractures in the elderly result from some form of trauma, usually a fall. Almost all of these fractures in elderly white women fall into this category. The most common sites for fractures due to a fall include the wrist, proximal radius—the forearm, the hip, the kneecap, the ankle, foot and toes, pelvis, face, lower leg bones including the tibia and fibula, and the ribs. Osteoporotic fractures result from minimal trauma, yet the forces that occur when elderly osteoporotic women fall are great enough to break normal healthy bones, so the term *minimal* may not be correct. Vertebral fractures in osteoporosis usually do not result from a fall or from any other obvious trauma. Traumatic fractures in women with osteoporosis usually affect the foot, toe, hand, fingers, and ribs, and the trauma is usually not a fall.

The whole process of falling and fracturing is somewhat complex. Several risk factors increase the risk of falling, including gait problems, balance problems, muscle weakness, visual problems, use of sedative drugs, and household hazards such as a broken step that results in an older person's losing his or her balance and falling. One of the most important risk factors is the use of sedative or psychoactive drugs. These medications (common ones include antianxiety drugs for example as Valium®, Librium®, and Xanax®) are mild sedatives that can make the user less alert than usual. The result is slowed motor function or loss of balance and a predisposition to falling. Many studies have reported an increased risk of falling with sedative use, especially antianxiety medications (in particular, Valium®, Librium®, Ativan®, Xanax®, and Serax®, and cyclic antidepressants (in particular, Elavil®, Prozac®, and Paxal®). Although we know that these medications increase the risk of fractures in the elderly, we have not determined that by *not* using these medications, falls in the elderly can be prevented and the number of resulting fractures reduced. However, a simple procedure such as reducing the use of sedatives in the elderly seems reasonable. Everything possible should be done to prevent the elderly from falling.

THE BIOMECHANICS OF FALLING

Nearly one-third of elderly persons fall at least once a year, but only about 5 percent of these falls result in a fracture. Since most falls do not result in a fracture, even in women with very low bone mass, this suggests that the way a person falls is a very important determinant of whether a fracture will result.

The risk of falling is low when you are 30 years of age and much higher when you are 70, but the risk of fracturing by falling is very high when you are 90. With age, changes in the way people fall probably account for the increase in hip fractures per fall. In older persons, such changes might include an increasing likelihood of an unprotected fall onto the hip bone, or trochanter, a weakening of protective arm response, and a loss of energy-absorbing soft tissue over the hip or the femur bone. In general, factors that increase the energy or force directed to the bone during a fall, such as the faller's height and weight, or a greater height of the fall, may all increase the risk of a fracture. By contrast, when energy or forces from the fall are absorbed from the soft tissues around a bone or from the impact surface, the risk of a fracture from a fall may decrease.

Recent studies show that fallers who suffered a hip fracture were much more likely to have fallen sideways compared to others who fell and did not have a fracture. Increased potential energy from the fall and greater height of the faller also increased the risk of hip fracture with a fall. On the other hand, landing on a hand or an object, a longer arm length, and padded impact surfaces were protective. When a faller landed heavily on the hip, decreased bone density there greatly increased the risk of hip fracture. At this time, we do not know if the amount of soft tissue padding around the hip influences the risk of hip fracture, regardless of bone mineral density. Recent studies have also found that middle-aged women who were tall had a much greater risk of fractures. A study of nursing home residents who wore protective hip padding showed far fewer hip fractures. Therefore, anything that dampens or lessens the force of impact of a fall, such as protective padding around the hip or an energy-absorbing floor covering in places where elderly individuals reside, may decrease the rate and risk of hip fractures.

Other than hip fractures, very little research has been done on the biomechanics of other types of fractures. Wrist fractures usually involve a fall onto an outstretched hand. Falls to the side generally do not result in a wrist fracture but are likely to cause a hip fracture. Therefore, it appears that the orientation of the fall and the site of the impact are very important factors in determining the kind of fracture that will occur after a fall.

Forces in the spine generated by activities such as lifting, stepping down from a curb, or coughing can be sufficient to cause a vertebral fracture. Other factors, such as degenerative disc disease in the spine or arthritis in the spine, kyphosis ("dowager's hump" due to osteoporotic compression fractures of the spine), and the distribution of body weight can all influence biomechanical forces in the spine and the risk of vertebral fractures. The influence of biomechanical forces on vertebral fractures in the spine is now being investigated, but results are not yet available.

A group of investigators have been following elderly white women for about 8 years. The study group consisted of about 9500 white women who were 65 years of age or older and had not had a previous hip fracture (Table 4.1). The investigators followed these women for over 4 years and talked with them every 4 months during that time. During the follow-up period, about 192 women had their first hip fracture that was not due to an automobile accident. The important risk factors for a hip fracture in these women included a maternal history of a hip fracture (this nearly doubled a woman's risk) and weight loss since the age of 25. The risk of a hip fracture was higher in women who had had another fracture of any type after age 50, were tall at age 25, rated their own health as fair or poor, had previous hyperthyroidism, had been treated with long-acting benzodiazepines or anticonvulsant drugs, drank large amounts of caffeinated beverages, or spent 4 hours or less per day on their feet. On the physical examination, factors that were found to increase the risk of a hip fracture in these women included an inability to rise from a chair without the use of the arms, poor depth perception, poor contrast sensitivity, and a rapid resting heart rate. The investigators also found that the risk of a hip fracture increased dramatically the more risk factors a woman had. For example, one risk factor may have increased the risk of a hip fracture only to 2.0, but five risk factors increased the risk to nearly 20 times that of a woman with no risk factors. This study was probably one of the first to show that the more risk factors for a hip fracture a woman has, the higher her risk of having such a fracture. This study also identified risk factors that a

Table 4.1. *The Risk of Hip Fractures in Elderly White Women*

Factors that increase the risk

Age, every 5 years*
Poor self-rated health
History of hyperthyroidism
Current use of sedatives or antianxiety drugs
Family history of hip fracture in mother*
Tall as a young adult*
Dementia*
High caffeine intake
On feet less than 4 hours per day
Muscle weakness
Poor visual depth perception
Poor visual contrast sensitivity
Resting pulse above 80 beats per minute
Any bone fracture after age 50*
Late menarche*
Low bone mass
Parkinson's disease
Little or no sunlight exposure
Low body weight
Smoking

Factors that appear to decrease the risk

Increase in weight since age 25
Walking for exercise
Tea consumption

Factors that do not appear to be associated with the risk

Hair color
Ancestry
Materal fracture other than the hip
Number of children breast fed
Natural menopause before age 45
Past cigarette smoking
Daily calcium intake

---

*Untreatable risk factors.
Source: Adapted from Cumming, S.R., Nevitt, M.C., Browner, W., et al. Risk factors for hip fractures in elderly white women. *New England Journal of Medicine* 332: 767–773, 1995.

woman and her physician could modify or change to prevent a fracture. For example, a change in a woman's eyeglass prescription could improve her depth perception and contrast sensitivity. Stopping the use of long-acting benzodiazepines reduced her risk of falling and fracturing the hip.

Additional risk factors for hip fractures identified in other studies

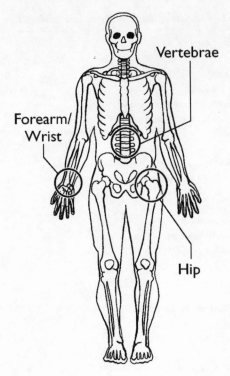

Figure 4.1 *The areas of the skeleton where osteoporotic fractures occur most often.*

include a history of falling, a fall in blood pressure when shifting from a sitting to a standing position or from a prone to a sitting position, use of four or more prescription drugs each day, little strength, poor flexibility, poor coordination, poor lower extremity sensations, poor balance, and recent hospitalization or other health-related activity restrictions.

HIP FRACTURES

The most severe osteoporotic fracture is the hip fracture, which typically results from falling while standing. It is usually painful and almost always requires hospitalization; for this reason, we know more about hip fractures than about any other type of osteoporotic fracture. Both men and women are at risk of fracturing a hip as they age. The average age of these patients is about 75 years. Most hip fractures result from a fall with a direct impact on the hip. The risk of hip fracture is lower if the person does not fall directly on the hip (Figure 4.1).

Hip fractures are very painful, but the pain is variable. In most patients the fracture is easy to diagnose because the patient is in pain, cannot rise from a chair, and cannot rotate the hip joint. The diagnosis is confirmed by X-ray. The two places in the hip bone, or femur, that break are the neck of the femur and the trochanteric area (see Figure 3.2). According to recent studies, trochanteric fractures are usually osteoporotic, and the risk of fractures increases with age. In general, patients with trochanteric hip fractures are about 5 years older than those with fractures at the neck of the femur.

Most femoral neck fractures require either surgery to pin the fracture or total joint replacement. Most trochanteric fractures are handled with pin surgery.

In osteoporotic patients fractures heal normally, but complications can occur. Depending in part on the patient's age and other medical problems, a hip fracture can mean hospitalization and a long recovery period. Problems that arise after the fracture are frequently due to difficulty in moving around either before or after the accident. And despite good surgery, about one-third of the women do not regain their former independence, and two-thirds require nursing home care. Only about one-quarter of women who fracture their hip regain their former mobility; over half need assistance with walking and everyday activities.

Some elderly patients develop complications, such as pneumonia, that prove fatal. In as many as one-third of the patients, the hip fracture sets in motion a cascade of other events resulting in death. Immobilization after the fracture, the surgery itself, and other medical problems can lead to complications. Women who fracture their hips tend to be less healthy than those who do not. Elderly women who fracture a hip have a nearly threefold higher risk of dying in the first year after the fracture than women of the same age with no fracture. In the second and third years after a hip fracture, the risk of dying levels off, suggesting that the first year after the fracture is the most dangerous.

VERTEBRAL FRACTURES

Vertebral fractures are another serious result of osteoporosis. They are classified by the shape of the vertebra after the fracture and are classified as central, wedge, or crush fractures—the last type involving the whole vertebra (Figure 4.2). These fractures occur spontaneously or as a result of very little trauma. They usually affect the area

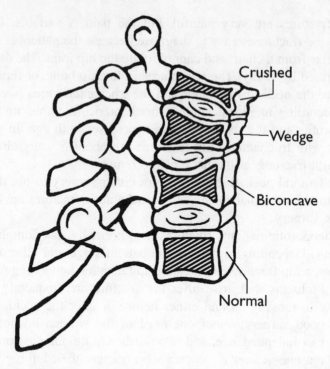

Figure 4.2 *The different types of vertebral fractures. Notice the normal vertebra; then observe the biconcave, or endplate, deformity, which results in compression of the middle of the endplate. The wedge fracture results from compression of the anterior, or front, part of the vertebra, and the total crush fracture results from compression of both the anterior, or front, and posterior, or back, sides of the vertebra. Vertebral fractures result in loss of height, and wedge fractures result in a kyphotic, or forward-bending, posture.*

from the midportion of the thoracic spine (the middle of the back behind the ribs) to the midportion of the lumbar spine (the lower back behind the abdomen). Almost half of the women who develop one vertebral fracture will eventually have another.

We do not know how many women develop vertebral fractures because many of these fractures do not cause pain and so do not come to the doctor's attention. Also, these fractures can cause back pain, and since back pain is common in many people, both young and old, we usually dismiss it.

With a fracture of the vertebrae, most of us experience back pain, a kyphosis (hump) that develops in the back, and loss of height. New back pain may be a signal of a new vertebral crush fracture. These fractures often occur while lifting, bending, coughing, or rising from a chair. They may occur suddenly or may develop a few days after an injury. The back pain usually radiates to the abdomen at the level at which the vertebra was fractured. The pain can increase with sitting or standing and is usually relieved by bed rest. Also, with coughing or sneezing, the pain can become quite severe, and a pain reliever will be necessary. Some women also complain of loss of appetite or abdominal fullness after vertebral fractures. Usually the pain decreases a few weeks after the fracture and may disappear completely. Some women may never have acute pain but will develop chronic low back pain after a fracture. Other women never have any complaints but notice a loss of height. Painless vertebral fracture is very rarely a cause of death, but more women with vertebral fractures die compared to those of the same age who do not.

A woman with one vertebral fracture has a very high risk of developing another. In one study that followed women for over 10 years, more than three-fourths of those with one vertebral fractures suffered another, and many of them lost more than 4 inches in height.

Multiple vertebral fractures increase the risk of developing a hump in the upper part of the back behind the rib cage. When the hump becomes noticeable, the following happens:

- The woman must hyperextend her neck to compensate, causing neck pain and muscle fatigue because she is using a different posture in which her chin nearly rests on the front of her rib cage.
- The hump reduces lung volume, preventing the lung from filling up with air.
- The hump reduces abdominal volume, causing the abdomen to protrude.
- The change in appearance may be very distressing, preventing the woman from dressing well and socializing.
- Often women with multiple fractures express a fear of falling and may limit their activities to those they feel comfortable doing.

FOREARM FRACTURES

Over 80 percent of forearm fractures occur in the distal radius (at the end of the bone, just before the wrist joint). They are referred to as *Colles' fractures*. They usually occur by falling on an outstretched hand. A woman's lifetime risk of having a Colles' fracture is about 15 percent. Although these fractures generally occur after menopause, they also occur in premenopausal women. This shows the importance of peak bone mass in determining a the risk of osteoporotic fracture. Forearm fractures are painful and usually require 4 to 6 weeks in a cast. The risk of developing a long-term complication after such a fracture increases with age. Some women do not recover immediate function, and there can be continued pain, tenderness, stiffness, swelling, and heat and cold disturbances of the hand for many months afterwards. Usually, after a year, only the stiffness is left. Compared to other osteoporotic fractures, some studies suggest that death rates are no higher in women with forearm fractures than in the general population.

ASSESSMENT OF FRACTURE RISK

Bone measurements are used to assess a woman's risk of developing an osteoporotic fracture. Many studies have shown that the risk of fracture increases as the bone mass decreases. For each standard deviation of below-peak bone mass, the fracture risk nearly doubles. A woman with a low bone mass can be given a lifetime fracture risk; that is, she can be told that a woman with a particular bone density has a certain lifetime risk of developing an osteoporotic fracture. The fracture may not occur for 20 years or it may happen in 5 years.

The bone site used to measure the bone mass can show the overall risk of developing an osteoporotic fracture both there and at other sites. In general, the prediction of a future fracture is more accurate if the doctor obtains a measurement at the site in question. For example, the risk of developing a vertebral fracture can be stated more confidently if the measurement is made at the spine. A bone mass measurement at the hip will predict a hip fracture more accurately than a measurement at another site.

SUMMARY

- Osteoporosis results in fractures, most often at the vertebrae, back, hip, and forearm or wrist.
- All fractures in elderly women, or in any person who has low bone mass, that result from low-force trauma are osteoporotic fractures.
- Hip fractures result from a fall. Risk factors for such fractures include low bone mass, older age, poor health, use of antianxiety

medications, a history of hip fracture in a mother or grandmother, muscle weakness, dementia, and sedentary lifestyle.

- Risk factors for fracture of the spine and forearm are less well characterized than those for fracture of the hip. Low bone mass and older age increase the risk.

5

Do Men Get Osteoporosis?

Osteoporosis in men has received much less attention than osteoporosis in women. This is too bad because recent studies have found that osteoporotic vertebral fractures occur more often in men than was previously thought, even though only half as many men as women are affected. Men suffer only 25 percent of all hip fractures, but the overall cost, the suffering endured, and resulting deaths are actually greater in men than in women. Since the elderly male population is increasing rapidly, osteoporosis will soon become a major health problem for many men.

Men were somewhat ignored in early studies of osteoporosis because osteoporotic fractures tend to occur at least 10 to 15 years later in men than in women. Men achieve a higher peak bone mass than women, so they have more bone to lose before they reach the point where the risk of fracture is high. Men's bones have a greater cross-sectional area and are larger in size. Also, aging men lose cortical bone more slowly than aging women do, and their pattern of bone loss is different.

When women go through menopause, estrogen deficiency results in increased bone turnover. When this happens, the number of trabeculae decreases as trabecular bone mass is lost. The result is a structural change that, over time, increases both bone fragility and the risk of fractures. In men, the pattern is different. Their trabeculae thin but do not disconnect or perforate, so the structure of their bone does not change much, and the bone does not become fragile as rapidly as it does in women. Of course, men do not go through menopause, so they do not have the accelerated loss of bone mass that occurs suddenly in women with the loss of estrogen. Aging men lose bone mass in a very slow, progressive manner. But men on average also have shorter lives than women, so the number of years they must withstand thin bones are fewer, and the risk of falling and fracturing their bones is much lower. Men also fall less than women do. So, while an elderly man's bone mass may be low, because he does not fall as often as an elderly woman, his risk of fracturing a hip is lower. However, age-related bone loss will, over time, result in osteoporosis in all men.

RISK FACTORS

There are many medical problems and disorders that can increase a man's risk of developing osteoporosis. These include the following:

- Several endocrine diseases have been linked to osteoporosis in men: hypogonadism (low levels of gonadal hormones, especially testosterone), Cushing's syndrome (elevated levels of steroids that thin bone), primary hyperparathyroidism (elevated parathyroid hormone, which increases bone resorption), acromegaly (too much growth hormone), hyperprolactinemia (too much circulating prolactin hormone), and hypercalciuria (too much calcium lost in the urine).
- Diseases that cause osteomalacia (problems with bone mineralization) include vitamin D deficiency, metabolic acidosis (a high acid level in the body), and other diseases that inhibit mineralization of bone.
- Cancers can lead to bone loss. The cancers seen in elderly men that might cause this include multiple myeloma (cancer of the bone marrow cells), and diseases that increase the number of white blood cells in the body and occasionally cause enlargement of lymph nodes.
- Some diseases involving an inherited defect in the type I collagen molecule (the major protein in bone) have also been linked to osteoporosis. Some of them are osteogenesis imperfecta, Ehlers-Danlos syndrome, Marfan's syndrome, and homocystinuria.
- Other conditions that can cause low bone mass in men include prolonged immobilization, a chronic inflammatory disease like rheumatoid arthritis, liver or kidney failure, and sarcoid (noninfectious, noncancerous enlargement of lymph nodes and other glands with inflammatory tissue).

Drugs that cause osteoporosis in women have the same effect in men. These include steroids, alcohol, too much thyroid hormone, chronic anticoagulation with heparin, antiseizure medications, and tobacco.

Probably the most common cause of osteoporosis in up to 30 percent of men is long-standing testosterone deficiency. While men usually detect a problem at about the age of 60, a low testosterone level, impotence, and decreased sex drive probably have existed for up to 20 years. Almost any cause of low testosterone may lead to osteoporosis in men. Testosterone deficiency is a significant risk factor for hip fracture in elderly men. It is probably also associated with the bone loss that accompanies aging in general, the bone loss associated with cancer and other chronic diseases, malnutrition, alcohol abuse, and excess steroids.

Hypogonadism in men is often hard to detect. The testes, which produce testosterone, can be normal in size, denial of symptoms is common, and men may have normal sexual function despite low testosterone. In general, men with osteoporosis should have their testosterone and luteinizing hormone (the hormone that stimulates the testes to make testosterone) measured.

Testosterone deficiency in men does not have the same effect on bone as estrogen deficiency does in postmenopausal women. In women, estrogen deficiency increases bone turnover, leading to greater bone resorption than bone formation and a net loss of bone. In men, testosterone deficiency also increases bone turnover but bone formation is below normal, resulting in a net loss of bone. The abnormalities in bone turnover in men with testosterone deficiency are correctable with testosterone replacement, just as the the abnormalities in bone turnover in women are correctable with estrogen replacement.

In men with osteoporosis, testosterone is normally converted to estrogen. Some of these men are unable to respond to the estrogen and become estrogen resistant. In men, the ability of bone cells to convert testosterone to estrogen may be critical in maintaining bone mineral density. More research is needed to better understand the balance between testosterone and estrogen and its relationship to bone mass in men.

IDIOPATHIC OR AGE-RELATED OSTEOPOROSIS IN MEN

Osteoporosis in men with no known cause is called *idiopathic* osteoporosis. This diagnosis should be made only after all other causes of osteoporosis have been ruled out. Idiopathic osteoporosis accounts for nearly half of the cases of osteoporosis in men. These men usually complain of back pain and have a vertebral compression fracture generally in their 50s or 60s. Unfortunately, as many as three or four compression fractures may have occurred before the patient goes to a doctor.

In men, bone mass is lost gradually at cortical bone sites (such as the forearm or hip); the loss ranges from 1 to 2 percent to up to 10 percent every decade after the age of 70. Cortical bone is lost from the inside bone surface, but it can be replaced at the outside surface, with no real reduction in cross-sectional bone area and no loss of bending strength with age. Trabecular bone loss is somewhat similar to that in women, with a loss of about 7 to 12 percent per decade. In women, there is only a slightly greater rate of loss in early menopause for about 5 years. But there are qualitative differences in the way men and women lose trabecular bone with age. Men tend to thin their trabeculae; women lose more trabeculae, which may disproportionately reduce the strength of their trabecular bone.

These are many reasons for age-related bone mass loss in men:

- Most important, osteoblast function decreases with age. Whether this is due to a shortened osteoblast life span or decreased osteoblast activity is not known.
- Older men spend less time exercising and remaining active, so they lose muscle mass, which may influence bone mass as well.
- Older men take in less calcium in their diet and their bodies absorb less calcium. This may also be related to insufficient vitamin D intake or intestinal resistance to the actions of vitamin D with age.
- Testosterone levels also fall off with age and may contribute to age-related bone loss.
- Falls increase with age, increasing the risk of fractures.

The risk factors for osteoporosis in men are summarized in Table 5.1.

HOW DO WE PREVENT OSTEOPOROSIS IN MEN?

Treatment for established osteoporosis in men is inadequate, and there is no therapy to prevent osteoporotic fractures. So, as in women, the emphasis is on prevention, focusing on ways to decrease bone loss (see Table 5.2).

Some of the preventive measures are very simple, including taking calcium and vitamin D supplements after the age of 60 or 65 years. Also important is regular low-impact physical activity three or four times a week, which helps maintain muscle mass and good balance and prevents further bone loss. Men should have an evaluation for

Table 5.1. *Risk Factors for Osteoporosis in Men*

White or Asian ancestry
Impaired gonadal function
Excessive alcohol use
Cigarette smoking
Medication use
   Steroids
   Anticonvulsants or antiseizure medications
   Thyroid hormone replacement
Chronic illness
Prolonged inactivity
Inactive lifestyle
Low dietary calcium intake
Lean body build
Family history of osteoporotic fractures
History of gastric or stomach surgery or intestinal resection

testosterone deficiency because this problem is easily correctable. They should also limit their alcohol intake to two or three drinks a day and avoid smoking because the nicotine in cigarettes decreases bone mass. Special programs are now being developed to prevent falls in the elderly; these may include such things as hip padding and special exercise programs.

There are no studies of medical treatments to prevent or reverse osteoporosis in men. Testosterone therapy is perhaps the best means of preventing further bone loss if the testosterone level is low. Antiresorptive agents, including bisphosphonates and calcitonin, will also probably help to prevent further bone loss in osteoporotic men. These drugs are discussed in Chapter 7. Studies are still needed to determine if these drugs will be as successful with men as they have been with women in preventing fractures.

SUMMARY

- Like women, men develop low bone mass and fractures; however, these conditions occur later in life (beginning at age 70).
- Men, like women, lose bone mass at the rate of about 1 percent per year from age 70 on.
- Lifestyle factors such as smoking and alcohol use, and medical problems such as low testosterone level and medication use, can also lower bone mass in men.

Table 5.2. *How to Prevent Osteoporosis in Men*

Calcium supplementation
   1000 milligrams a day in younger men and preadolescent boys
   1500 milligrams a day in adolescent boys and men older than 60 years of age
Vitamin D intake of 600 to 800 IU per day in men older than 60
Lifelong regular physical activity
Early recognition and treatment of testosterone deficiency
Limited alcohol intake and no cigarette smoking
Avoidance of falls

- Treatment to prevent osteoporosis in men is not as well developed as it is for women.
- Preventive measures include calcium and vitamin D supplementation in elderly men, testosterone replacement if indicated, and reduction of smoking and alcohol intake. Other treatments, including bisphosphonates and calcitonin, also help to prevent bone loss in men.

Part II
PREVENTION AND TREATMENT OF OSTEOPOROSIS

6

Prevention of Osteoporosis and Management of Menopause with Hormone Replacement Therapy

Prevention of osteoporosis means prevention of low bone mass. Since bone mass at any age, at least until the age of 75, depends largely on the peak bone mass obtained at age 30, prevention should focus on anything that can increase peak bone mass. The problem is that the major determinants of peak bone mass are unchangeable, and the value of factors such as nutrition and exercise is uncertain. Even if we could identify, at the age of 13 or earlier, girls who are destined to become osteoporotic and those who will fracture, we probably could not persuade them to change their lifestyle or accept a therapy to prevent a disease from occurring 50 years later. Also, although we believe that lifestyle factors are important in determining bone mass and rates of osteoporotic fractures, we are not sure that lifestyle changes will prevent osteoporosis. For these reasons and others, prevention is focused on preventing the bone loss that occurs with menopause, when osteoporosis is diagnosed, or when an individual becomes inactive and risks developing osteoporosis. Most of the interventions involve hormones.

HOW DO HORMONES PREVENT OR TREAT OSTEOPOROSIS?

Hormone replacement therapy (HRT) involves the use of estrogen, either alone or in combination with progesterone hormones. HRT is given to replace the body's estrogen after menopause. Because estrogen used alone involves the risk of uterine and other cancers, progestins have been added to recent formulations. Progestins, taken either together with estrogen or on alternative days, usually remove the risk of developing uterine cancer. But it is very important for a woman to know what combination of hormones she is receiving and to understand her own risk of cancer based on her family history.

Hormone replacement therapy will prevent bone loss at menopause that stems from estrogen deficiency and for many years thereafter. This arrest in bone loss will last as long as estrogen treatment continues, at least until the age of 70 and maybe beyond. When estrogen is stopped, bone loss recurs at the rate occurring before the estrogen treatment. For a woman to take full advantage of the bone-sparing effects of HRT, she should start therapy as soon as possible after menopause. Studies consistently show that HRT reduces the risk of osteoporotic fractures of the hip and the forearm by about 30 to 40 percent and the risk of fractures of the spine by over 50 percent. The longer a woman takes estrogen after menopause, the lower her risk of suffering an osteoporotic fracture.

HOW LONG MUST I STAY ON HRT?

Women who start HRT at menopause and continue it for 7 to 10 years will gain long-term protection against an osteoporotic fracture. But menopause usually begins between 50 and 54 years of age, and generally fractures do not begin until after the age of 70. So, if a woman takes HRT from age 54 to age 64 and then stops, what will happen to the bone that she has maintained or preserved? Most studies show that this bone is not rapidly lost when treatment stops. In one study of women who were treated with HRT for 4 years who stopped taking it for 6 years, bone mass was found to decrease by only 10 percent, or less than 2 percent a year. Moreover, in women who were followed up to 10 years after stopping treatment, bone mass decreased by 20 percent. So we conclude that the amount of bone mass saved by taking HRT for 4 years persisted for at least 6 years and probably even longer.

How long should women stay on HRT? This is controversial because of the uncertainties regarding the long-term risks and benefits. Women should discuss the risks and benefits of this treatment with their physician. Each woman is different, with different risks and a different personal history. So, no one recommendation is appropriate for all. Ten years of treatment is considered optimal to protect against bone loss and to prevent osteoporotic fractures. We will need to wait another 10 years to be sure that longer treatments can be safely recommended.

ARE THERE OTHER RISKS AND BENEFITS OF HRT?

These days, not a week goes by without a newspaper article that reports the benefits or risks of HRT. And since the population of aging women is larger now than ever, with a good chance that most women will live well into their 80s, the issues surrounding women's health will become more and more urgent. At the forefront is the great debate about the risk of HRT, and the discussion has become heated and divided.

Estrogen and Heart Disease

There is no doubt and little debate about estrogen's beneficial effect on coronary artery disease. The incidence or risk of coronary heart disease is very low in premenopausal women, but as women age, the risk progressively increases, approaching that of men. We do not know the exact process involved.

Estrogen therapy decreases the risk of heart disease in women by about 30 to 50 percent. The dose of estrogen used in most of the studies on this subject is between 0.625 and 1.25 milligrams of *conjugated estrogens* (a mixture of estrogens from natural sources) (Premarin ®) a day. Unfortunately, at this time we do not know how long a woman must take estrogen to obtain this effect.

Estrogen probably protects against heart disease by reducing cholesterol, a very strong risk factor for heart disease. Estrogen appears to reduce total cholesterol and low density lipoprotein (LDL, the bad cholesterol) and to increase high density lipoprotein (HDL, the good cholesterol). And the higher the dose of estrogen, the greater the reduction in LDL and the greater the increase in HDL.

Progestins, hormones made in the ovaries, are frequently given to women who have not had a hysterectomy and take estrogen. Since estrogen therapy can cause the layer of cells lining the uterus (or endometrium) to grow, progestins allow the uterus to shed these cells, which results in a menstrual period. To protect the uterus from possible problems with estrogen use, progestins are given in conjunction with estrogen. Some studies suggest that progestins lessen the beneficial effects of estrogen on HDL and LDL, and possibly on heart disease as well. In general, progestins are used intermittently or daily at a very low dose so that they appear to have no long-term effect on lipid levels.

Since the number one cause of death in elderly women is heart disease, there is a good reason for a woman going through menopause to consider HRT, especially if she has a strong family history of heart disease. If a woman has a strong family history of heart disease or many significant risk factors, estrogen therapy may prolong her life.

The Risk of Endometrial Cancer

It is clear that the woman who uses estrogen alone for a long time runs an increased risk of developing cancer of the endometrium. The risk in women who have used estrogen alone, compared to women who have never used estrogen, is about two times higher. This effect increases with the number of years of therapy and with higher doses of estrogen. The addition of a progestin, which causes shedding of the endometrium, prevents this increased endometrial cancer risk provided that the dose and the schedule of progestin treatment can prevent endometrial *hyperplasia* (thickening of the cells in the lining of the uterus).

Today there are many different treatments that include a progestin. Some women take a progestin every day with the estrogen. Others take progestin for 10 days a month and estrogen for 30 days. Still others take progestin for only 10 days every 3 months. The time schedule and dose of the progestin depend on each woman's response to the estrogen treatment. For example, some women have more endometrial hyperplasia than others on estrogen and need to take progestin every month for 10 days to completely shed the endometrial lining. In other women, estrogen will have almost no effect on the endometrial lining; and these women may need only a progestin for 10 days every 3 months. Finally, some women prefer to take both medications every day. The progestin is given at a lower dose, so they never experience thickening of the uterine wall and the shedding resembling a menstrual period. Preventing endometrial cancer by adding a progestin is simple. How each woman adapts to the new medication and how often she needs to take the progestin is individual. You will need to ask your physician about your risk and work out a treatment schedule you can both live with.

The Risk of Breast Cancer

Does estrogen treatment increase a woman's risk of developing breast cancer? Over 40 studies since 1970 have examined this issue, but the findings are inconsistent. Some of the studies followed women who took estrogen for over 10 to 15 years and found a small increase in risk. A more recent study found that 15 years of estrogen use might increase the risk of breast cancer by about 1.5 times compared to the risk of a woman who has never taken estrogen. Another recent study of nurses found that the risk of breast cancer increased as women aged, and that the longer a woman took estrogen, the higher the risk. Yet the increased risk of breast cancer in the group of women older than 65 who had taken estrogen for over 10 years was only 1.7 times as great. Therefore, the risk of breast cancer increases with age in women, whether they take estrogen or not. Moreover, as women age and the longer they take estrogen, the risk of breast cancer may also increase, but the increase is quite small.

An important point to add to this discussion is that when breast cancer does develop in women taking estrogen, it need not be fatal. We can interpret this to mean that the risk of developing breast cancer is probably established early in life, and it may also be genetically determined. While HRT may accelerate breast cancer in some women, others may not be at risk, either with or without this therapy. However, this is only a guess.

The real risk of breast cancer in women taking estrogen is probably small, just over 1 to 1.5 times the risk of women who are not on estrogen. Over the next few years, more information from ongoing studies will help us better determine the real risk of breast cancer with estrogen use.

The Risk of Stroke

There is some evidence that estrogen decreases the risk of a stroke. But at this time, there is no definite information regarding the effect of estrogen or progestins on the risk of stroke in women.

Estrogen and Dementia

There is now some very early evidence that regular long-term estrogen use may prevent the development of dementia in older women. A recent study of women living in a retirement community in Southern California found that those who took estrogen had a nearly 35 percent lower risk of developing Alzheimer's disease or dementia compared to nonusers of the same age. It appears that the risk was reduced with almost all types of estrogen preparations, including pills, creams, and injections. The risk of Alzheimer's disease decreased the higher the dose of estrogen and the longer it was taken. This was one of the first studies to show that estrogen may be useful for preventing or delaying the onset of dementia in postmenopausal women.

ESTROGEN THERAPY AND THE MANAGEMENT OF MENOPAUSE

The management of menopause is beyond the scope of this book and involves more than a prescription for HRT. The main purpose of menopause treatment is to provide relief from acute symptoms including hot flashes, vaginal dryness, mood swings, dry skin, loss of sex drive, loss of flexibility, and weight gain. But recently, the medical community has begun to try to prevent some of the long-term complications from menopause or estrogen deficiency, including coronary artery disease, colon cancer, and osteoporosis. Thus, when a woman goes through menopause, her physician will probably assess both the acute symptoms of menopause and her risk of developing cardiovascular disease or osteoporosis. The dose and duration of HRT chosen will depend on the goals of the treatment.

Acute Menopausal Symptoms

Acute menopausal symptoms mostly result from reduced estrogen levels in the bloodstream. The most dreaded of the acute menopausal symptoms are hot flashes. If you are bothered by hot flashes, you can treat them in many different ways. You can wait a while, as hot flashes decrease over time; you can try natural remedies like keeping your environment cool and not overdressing; and you can keep your caffeine and alcohol intake low. If natural remedies do not work, you can try HRT.

HRT relieves most of the symptoms due to estrogen deficiency, including hot flashes. Usually hot flashes and night sweats improve after about 2 weeks of treatment, and the maximum effect is usually seen by 3 months. If menopausal symptoms still occur, the dose of the estrogen can be increased or another type of estrogen or an alternative medication can be tried. The severity of the menopausal symptoms is believed to be related to the fluctuations in gonadal hormone levels. These fluctuations gradually decrease over several years, and the hot flashes stop completely or become less common. For this reason, HRT is frequently stopped after a few years when the symptoms are not likely to recur.

For women who cannot or will not take estrogen, other treatments for hot flashes are available. Progestins can control both hot flashes and night sweats. Hypnotics, sedatives, and tranquilizers are also used to reduce hot flashes, but they do not relieve other menopausal symptoms and can make a woman feel very tired. Vaginal dryness, another symptom of estrogen deficiency, can result in painful intercourse. This can be treated with moisturizers or vaginal creams with estrogen.

Are There Any Risks or Contraindications in Taking HRT?

There are very few contraindications—conditions that rule out estrogen therapy. Some people think that a woman's age should determine whether she takes estrogen, but the risks and benefits of therapy do not change with age; HRT appears to prevent osteoporosis just as well at the age of 70 as at the age of 50. One drawback to HRT is the reappearance of menstrual periods. Some women find this to be a problem; it may be helped somewhat by continuous daily use of an estrogen and a progestin.

Several contraindications are listed in the estrogen product information brochure that accompanies the prescription, but these should be interpreted very carefully. Drug companies obtained this information by using high doses of synthetic estrogens that were used in early birth control pills. These contraindications include high blood pressure, a previous heart attack, a family history of heart disease, varicose veins, a history of a blood clot or phlebitis, preexisting gallstones, and heavy smoking. Recent evidence shows that HRT is particularly beneficial in women with heart disease. Other contraindications sometimes listed include obesity, a history of melanoma (a skin cancer), previously abnormal cervical cells, gallstones, previous cervical or ovarian cancer, surgery occurring at the time of HRT therapy, and a family history of breast cancer. There is very little evidence that these conditions should be considered contraindications to HRT.

But there are several conditions a physician should weigh carefully before starting HRT. These conditions do not mean a woman cannot take HRT; it means her physician will need to monitor her condition closely during therapy. If these conditions worsen, the therapy should be stopped. The conditions include uncontrolled high blood pressure, migraine headaches, a previous blood clot in the legs or lung, diabetes, preexisting gallstones, mild liver disease, endometriosis, and uterine fibroids.

But there are several conditions that will prevent you from taking estrogen therapy. These include endometrial cancer or breast cancer in you or two of your first-degree relatives, undiagnosed abnormal vaginal bleeding, and severe active liver disease with abnormalities on liver function tests. Another important consideration is that melanoma, a form of skin cancer, may recur more rapidly during pregnancy and HRT treatment. For this reason, any woman with a history of melanoma should avoid HRT if there is a significant chance that it will recur.

THE MANY TYPES OF ESTROGEN THERAPY

Many different forms of estrogen are used for HRT, and they go by many names. Some of the most common are 17 beta estradiol and its derivatives; estrone, estriol, and conjugated estrogens (Premarin®) isolated from a pregnant mare's urine. Today HRT is available in many forms. The most common form is a pill or tablet. Some women prefer a skin patch, which is convenient, inexpensive, and easily stopped if necessary. Skin estrogen patches are similar to the popular nicotine patches now on the market. Some forms of HRT used to prevent and treat osteoporosis are listed in Table 6.1.

Combination Therapies

Some physicians prescribe estrogen as well as a progestin for women who have not had a hysterectomy. This type of therapy is called *opposed estrogen therapy* because the progestin helps to manage the potentially risky side effects of estrogen. When the progestin is stopped, menstrual periods recur; this is a common reason women stop taking HRT.

Progestins are classified and named according to the number of carbon atoms they contain. The C-21 progestins are generally used for HRT because they seem to have fewer side effects and do not raise the cholesterol level. Progestins can be given daily at a low dose with estrogen. Combination preparations are now available or are given for only the last 10 days of the menstrual cycle. In general, a physician will tailor the dose and duration of progestin therapy to the patient's needs.

Side effects do occur. Women on cyclical progestins commonly

Table 6.1. *Examples of HRTs Approved for the Prevention and Treatment of Osteoporosis*

Drug	Composition	Dosage
Premarin	Estrogen	0.625 milligrams/day
Prempro	Estrogen*	
	Medroxyprogesterone acetate	0.625 milligrams/day
		2.5 milligrams/day
Premphase	Estrogen	0.625 milligram/day
	Medroxyprogesterone acetate	5 milligrams/day
Ogen	Estrogen	0.625 milligram/day
Estrace	Estrogen	0.5 milligram/day
Estraderm	Estrogen	0.05 milligram twice a week
Climora Transdermal	Estrogen	0.05 milligram/day by patch once a week
		0.1 milligram per day transdermally

*Generic preparations are approved for many prescriptions.
Source: Adapted from Greenwood, S. *Menopause, Naturally* (Updated). Volcano, CA: Volcano Press, 1992.

complain of a feeling of fullness or bloating, which can often be relieved by changing to another progestin. Other side effects include headaches, breast soreness, mood changes, and acne.

Side effects of estrogens include fluid retention, breast soreness, and headaches. Other side effects include nausea, leg cramps, upper abdominal fullness or dyspepsia, and heavy bleeding when menstrual periods resume with cyclic progestin treatment. Most women who stay on estrogen lose weight. After many years of estrogen use, total body fat also decreases.

Combined Continuous HRT

Today many combined estrogen progestin therapies are available (see Table 6.2). These medications seem to work best for postmenopausal women who wish to avoid or cannot tolerate withdrawal bleeding. These pills generally do not cause cyclical bleeding because the continuous progestin prevents the monthly thickening and shedding of the endometrial lining. Still, about 20 percent of women who take a combination pill will experience irregular bleeding for the first few months. Sometimes this can be minimized by increasing the dose of the progestin if the estrogen and progestin are taken separately. The combination treatment does not adversely affect cholesterol. The cholesterol levels are the same as those seen with estrogen treatment alone: HDL cholesterol goes up and LDL and total cholesterol decrease.

Table 6.2. *Use of Progestins in Combined HRT*

Composition	Dosage
	Cyclic
Medroxyprogesterone acetate	5–10 milligrams for days 1–14 of each month
Norethindrone	2.5 milligrams for days 1–14 each month
Natural progesterone	100 milligrams in a.m. and 200 milligrams in p.m. for days 1–14 each month
	Continuous—combined with estrogen
Medroxyprogesterone acetate	2.5–5 milligrams daily
Norethindrone	1 milligram daily
Natural progesterone	100 milligrams twice daily

Source: Adapted from Greenwood, S. *Menopause, Naturally* (Updated). Volcano, CA: Volcano Press 1992.

Other Types of Hormone Delivery Systems

Skin Patches

Estrogen can be given through the skin with the use of a patch that continuously releases estrogen into the bloodstream. The side effects of this delivery system are few. Sometimes women complain of headaches or skin irritation at the site of the patch. But a patch bypasses the liver, so the effects on cholesterol and lipids may be less with a patch compared to a pill or tablet. Women who have gallstones or liver problems may benefit from this method. Also, women who smoke should use the estrogen patch because smokers derive no benefit from oral estrogens since they break it down too fast. And because the patch system is so easy and lasts for 4 days, compliance may improve in women who have trouble taking pills daily.

Topical Creams

Topical estrogen vaginal creams relieve vaginal dryness and atrophic vaginitis (poor or low cell lining in the vagina). They are probably not an efficient way to deliver estrogen into the bloodstream because the absorption of estrogen from the vagina varies. If a woman uses only vaginal estrogen cream, a progestin is probably unnecessary as not enough estrogen enters her bloodstream to induce menstrual periods. Commonly used topical creams are listed in Table 6.3.

Table 6.3. *Commonly Used Estrogen Vaginal Creams*

Brand Name	Generic Name	Strength (per gram of cream)
Ogen cream	Estropipate or estrone	1.5 milligrams
Premarin cream	Conjugated estrogen	0.625 milligram
Estrace cream	Estradiol	0.1 milligram

Note: Additional creams are available at pharmacies, so consult your pharmacist or physician. Also, check with your physician or pharmacist about the dose needed.
Source: Adapted from Greenwood, S. *Menopause, Naurally* (Updated). Volcano, CA: Volcano Press, 1992.

TAMOXIFEN AND RALOXIFENE: ESTROGEN LOOKALIKES, AGONISTS, AND ANTAGONISTS (SELECTIVE ESTROGEN RECEPTOR MODULATORS [SERMS])

Recently, great interest has been generated by tamoxifen, an estrogen-like compound (selective estrogen receptor modulator, SERM) that has some properties of estrogen but without some of the negative side effects. For example, tamoxifen is used in women with breast cancer; it acts like an antiestrogen in breast tissue but like estrogen in other parts of the body. If a woman has a breast tumor that has been removed and the tumor cells have a protein on their surface (an *estrogen receptor*) that attaches to the tumor and stimulates cell growth, such tissue is called receptor-positive. Since estrogen may have stimulated the breast tissue to grow, in women who have estrogen-receptor positive breast tumors, tamoxifen acts as an antiestrogen, preventing this type of breast tumor from growing and spreading. Some studies show that this antiestrogen or SERM in the breast prevents recurrence of the cancer and the development of new cancers. Tamoxifen also has very weak estrogen activity in the uterus, so continued use results in very little endometrial or uterine cell growth. However, a small number of women develop abnormal uterine cell growth (hyperplasia), so women on tamoxifen must be followed carefully. Tamoxifen is a proestrogen or has estrogen-like properties in the bone and liver. So tamoxifen treatment in postmenopausal women, like estrogen treatment, prevents bone loss in the hip and spine. Moreover, tamoxifen lowers LDL cholesterol and raises HDL cholesterol. In summary, tamoxifen acts like estrogen in the bone and the liver but not in the breast and has fewer effects in the uterus. Because of these properties, other estrogen lookalikes or selective estrogen receptor modulators are being developed to prevent and treat osteoporosis. These compounds include raloxifene, droloxifene, and idoxifene. They target the tissues we want the estrogen to act on and bypass others where the effect could be harmful (such as breast tissue). Raloxifene has recently been approved by the Food and Drug Administration for the prevention of postmenopausal bone loss. In postmenopausal women, it prevents bone loss and does not cause uterine cell growth (hyperplasia); it also modestly reduces LDL cholesterol and increases HDL cholesterol. Early animal and clinical studies suggest that it has no effect on breast tissue. In fact, raloxifene may lower the risk of breast cancer.

The exciting news about these estrogen-like compounds or SERMs, is that they may allow us to treat women with a medication that provides all the benefits of estrogen without the negative side effects. More of these medications may be approved by the Food and Drug Administration in the near future.

One thing these estrogen-like compounds do not do is to control hot flashes that most women experience in the first few years of menopause. Therefore, in the future, a woman may take estrogen for the first few years of menopause until the hot flashes are controlled and then switch to an estrogen-like compound like raloxifene. The risk of breast cancer with estrogen use appears to increase with use, so using estrogen for 3 to 5 years of menopause will not increase the risk. The estrogen-like compounds (or SERMs) could then be taken for the rest of a woman's life to prevent bone loss and possibly heart disease without the fear of breast or uterine cancer.

HOW ARE PHYTOESTROGENS DIFFERENT FROM HRT MEDICATIONS?

Phytoestrogens are natural estrogens found in numerous plants. Soybeans and flaxseed, for example, have a high concentration of these estrogens. Phytoestrogens have a chemical structure similar to that of the estrogen in our bodies. They appear to have weak estrogen-like effects in preventing bone loss and heart disease, and they may have weak antiestrogen effects on breast tissue; thus, they may reduce the potential cancer risk from prolonged estrogen use. Some women report that taking phytoestrogens from soy milk and flaxseed decreases hot flashes and vaginal dryness. While there is growing interest in the use of estrogens derived from plants and vegetables, more research must be done before we know if they are different from the current estrogen medications. Phytoestrogen supplements can be obtained from health food stores, as well as from soy milk and flaxseed. Any woman who is interested in taking these supplements should discuss it with her doctor.

IF HRT IS SO GOOD, WHY DON'T WOMEN STAY ON IT?

Today the benefits of HRT are well known. The major problem is that many women are reluctant to take it. If it is started at the beginning of menopause and if women fail to take it long enough, they will not prevent osteoporosis and heart disease.

An estimated 20 to 50 percent of women start HRT at menopause in the United States and Europe; the rates in other countries are much lower. We do not know how many women stay on it for 5 to 10 years, the minimum time required to prevent osteoporotic fractures; the best estimate is less than 40 percent. On a more positive note, women treated daily with both estrogen and progestin, avoiding monthly menstrual periods, usually remained on the therapy for a few years. This is good news for women who need hormone replacement but dread the return of menstrual periods.

Fortunately, through public interest and education, the benefits of HRT are changing women's minds, and the number of prescriptions for HRT is increasing every year. Now we must watch to see if the women who start HRT stay on it long enough to reap the benefits and reduce the risk of developing osteoporotic fractures.

SUMMARY

- Prevention of osteoporosis means prevention of low bone mass. At menopause, estrogen levels decline about 50 percent and bone loss begins.
- Hormone replacement therapy (HRT) will prevent bone loss, reduce hot flashes, lower cholesterol to prevent heart disease, maintain vaginal lubrication, help to prevent dementia, possibly improve memory, promote a sense of well-being, and prevent colon cancer.
- HRT beginning at menopause and continuing for 7 to 10 years gives long-term protection against osteoporotic fractures.
- As with any type of medication, there are risks with HRT. The risk of breast cancer, other cancers, clotting problems, and gallstones must be carefully evaluated and discussed with one's doctor before beginning HRT.
- Combination HRT is now available to manage the potentially risky side effects of estrogen. These therapies too have side ef-

fects, including fluid retention, breast soreness, nausea, leg cramps, stomach fullness, and heavy menstrual bleeding.

- Hormones can also be taken via skin patches and vaginal creams.
- Tamoxifen and raloxifene are compounds that have some of the properties of estrogen without some of the side effects and can prevent osteoporosis and possibly breast cancer in high risk individuals.
- Phytoestrogens are natural estrogens found in foods such as soybeans and flaxseed. Their effects on prevention of osteoporosis are not known.

DEBRA: A CASE OF EARLY MENOPAUSE

Debra is a 30-year-old white woman, 5 feet 7 inches tall, weighing 120 pounds. At the age of 28, she experienced early menopause after a hysterectomy in which both ovaries were removed due to chronic pelvic pain from scarring, the result of endometriosis (uterine tissue growing outside the uterus). Debra was started on 0.625 milligram of Premarin®, a conjugated estrogen, 1 month after surgery. She has one child who was born when Debra was 20, and her mother is now 55 years old. Her two grandmothers are 70 and 65 years of age, and neither one has osteoporosis. Debra smokes a couple of cigarettes a day and drinks about five cups of coffee. Her daily calcium intake is nearly 1500 milligrams, and her vitamin D intake is 400 IU. She also walks briskly for exercise four times a week for nearly 1 hour.

When Debra's bone mineral content was measured, the bone mineral density of her spine was 0.88 g/cm², and her T score was +1.0.

Removal of her ovaries greatly increased Debra's risk of developing osteoporosis since she lost her natural estrogen before achieving her peak bone mass. This would result in rapid loss of bone mass, just as if she were going through the early years of menopause. Despite Debra's high risk of developing osteoporosis, her spinal bone mineral density 2 years after surgery is normal—probably because she was given estrogen replacement therapy almost immediately after surgery, so she has never experienced estrogen deficiency or the resulting loss of bone. Also, Debra has enough calcium, vitamin D, and exercise, all of which may have helped her maintain good bone mass.

But because Debra uses estrogen replacement therapy regularly, there are other risks for which she must be monitored. Most important, chronic estrogen therapy may involve a very small risk of breast cancer. Therefore, Debra must learn to perform manual breast self-examinations routinely and must have a mammogram every 2 years while she is on therapy to monitor for breast cancer. Because her uterus has been removed, Debra does not need to take a low dose of a progestin, which is prescribed to minimize the risk of uterine cancer.

How long will Debra need to take estrogen to prevent bone loss? We do not know, but we do know that if she stops taking it, a rapid loss of bone mass will occur. Debra will probably need to take estrogen for the rest of her life. If for some reason she cannot do so, another medication will have to be used. These alternative medications are discussed in Chapter 7.

Although Debra now has normal bone mass, as time passes she may lose bone mass while on the estrogen replacement therapy. Therefore, perhaps every 3 or 5 years, her bone mineral density should be checked again to be sure that the estrogen therapy is working. If she is losing bone mass, a higher dose of the estrogen may be needed or another medication may have to be added.

The ability to use estrogen replacement immediately after hysterectomy prevents the development of premature osteoporosis. This therapy is a safe and effective treatment, but physician follow-up is necessary to be sure that breast examinations are done to prevent breast cancer. Bone mineral density should also be measured periodically to be sure that bone mass is being maintained with the estrogen.

LAURIE: A FAMILY HISTORY OF OSTEOPOROSIS

Laurie is a 49-year-old white woman, 5 feet 8 inches tall, weighing 130 pounds. She has two children, started menstruating at age 14, and has generally had a normal menstrual cycle. She has a family history of osteoporosis; both her grandmother and her maternal aunt suffered vertebral compression fractures in their 70s. Laurie stopped menstruating about 1 year ago and has come in for an evaluation of her bone mineral density to determine if she needs medication to prevent or treat osteoporosis.

Laurie took birth control pills from age 20 to age 35. She does not smoke and drinks only a glass or two of wine a week. She eats a regular diet and exercises about once a week. Her usual calcium intake from her diet is about 700 milligrams a day; she does not take any vitamins. Her vitamin D intake is about 200 IU a day.

When her bone mineral density was measured in her lumbar spine, it was 0.77 g/cm^2 and her T score was -2.5.

Testing shows that Laurie has very low bone density, and even though she has not yet had an osteoporotic fracture, her lifetime risk is very high. The reasons for her low bone mass are probably genetic. She did not achieve a high peak bone mass at maturity. Now, at the start of menopause, she will lose more bone mass and further increase her risk of developing a fracture.

Prevention of bone loss is critical. First, Laurie must increase her daily intake of calcium through diet and a supplement to bring it up to 1500 milligrams a day. It would be best to get half of the calcium from a calcium carbonate supplement and half from her diet. Laurie should also take two multiple vitamins to increase her daily vitamin D intake to about 800 IU. She will also need a medication to prevent bone loss. Estrogen is the best choice if Laurie has no family history of breast cancer or intolerance to the medication. Estrogen should be combined with a progestin to prevent possible uterine cancer. If a progestin is given either daily or cyclically (for a few days each month) together with the estrogen, there is no increased risk of uterine cancer. Since Laurie will take two medications, she must see her primary care physician every year. The physician must do a uterine biopsy to check for uterine cell changes, and at least every other year a mammogram should be done to check for any breast changes while she is on estrogen. Laurie is responsible for making sure that everything is done to prevent the unwanted side effects of estrogen.

Estrogen therapy for postmenopausal women has the benefits of preventing heart disease, bone loss, and vaginal dryness, as well as decreasing hot flashes; it even may prevent dementia (such as Alzheimer's disease). Yet, prolonged use is associated with a slightly higher risk of breast cancer. Therefore, if a woman decides to take estrogen, she must also have an annual medical checkup to prevent any unwanted side effects.

Laurie decided to start estrogen therapy to prevent further bone loss. Now, in early menopause, her bone turnover is high, that is, she will lose more bone mass than she will from estrogen deficiency. Replacing lost estrogen will make her bone turnover normal again, and she should not lose more bone. But Laurie already has very low bone mass, or osteoporosis without a fracture, and may wonder if estrogen treatment is enough.

A few more options are open to Laurie today. Other groups of medications, called *bisphosphonates* and *calcitonin* (see Chapter 7), are available to treat osteoporosis. These drugs can prevent and even increase bone mass somewhat. Since Laurie has very low bone mass at menopause, she may decide, with her doctor, to start using one of them along with estrogen. However, the use of antiresorptive agents in combination to increase bone mass and reduce fractures is only experimental at this time (not approved by the FDA for treatment of osteoporosis).

How should Laurie's bone mass be monitored? After taking estrogen, calcium, and vitamin D for about 1 year, she should have another bone mineral density measurement to see if the estrogen is working. A year from now, Laurie should have either the same bone mass or a little more, about 1 to 3 percent more than when she first started the therapy. If it has stayed the same or increased, her doctor may continue to use this therapy. But if she has lost bone mass, another medication will probably have to be added to prevent further bone loss.

JUDY: ENTERING MENOPAUSE

Judy is a 54-year-old white woman who began menopause about 1 year ago. She is experiencing hot flashes once or twice a day. She has had very good health throughout her life and had two normal pregnancies. She has maintained a healthy diet and has exercised twice a week for the past 20 years. Her current height is 5 feet 7 inches, and she weighs 135 pounds. All of her grandparents and both parents lived well into their 80s, and there is no history of osteoporosis in any of her relatives. But Judy's father and mother both had heart disease beginning at about the age of 60, and Judy has a slightly high total cholesterol level of 250. Currently, her only medication is one multiple vitamin a day.

Judy's bone mineral density of the lumbar spine measures 1.2 g/cm^2 and her T score is +1.1. The bone mineral density of the femoral neck of the hip measures 1.2 g/cm^2, and the T scores is +1.7.

A bone mineral density scan shows that Judy has very high bone mineral density in both her spine and her hips, and her current risk of developing osteoporosis is low. At this time, a preventive medication may not be necessary. On the other hand, Judy has risk factors for cardiovascular disease, and for that reason alone, she should consider starting estrogen replacement therapy. This therapy in postmenopausal women reduces the risk of heart disease by over 30 percent. It will also reduce or completely eliminate her hot flashes. Judy should also obtain information about starting a low-fat, low-cholesterol diet.

How long must Judy stay on estrogen therapy to reap the benefits for her heart? We are not sure. The length of time hot flashes last is variable—usually about 5 years. On the other hand, the risk of heart disease will continue or increase for the rest of her life. Judy may need to stay on estrogen for life, and as she grows older, she may also need to add another medication to lower her cholesterol.

Since Judy is now postmenopausal, she will need to increase her calcium intake to about 1500 milligrams a day. She will obtain enough vitamin D with her multiple vitamin and by being out in sunlight once a day. Her current exercise program is adequate to maintain her bone mass and cardiovascular fitness.

Since Judy has very high bone mass for her age and a very low risk of developing osteoporosis, she probably will not need a repeat bone mineral density scan for several years. As another way to monitor her bone changes, her doctor can order blood and urine tests that would reveal Judy's bone turnover. If these tests are done before she starts estrogen therapy, and again a few months afterward, her doctor can tell if estrogen is preserving her bone mass. Monitoring of bone turnover through blood and urine tests is beginning to be used in doctors' practices today, and in a few years it may replace the more costly bone mineral density test.

GEORGIA: LOW BONE MASS AT 75 YEARS OF AGE AND HIGH CHOLESTEROL

Georgia is a 75-year-old white woman who is 5 feet 4 inches tall and weighs 130 pounds. She has been in good health all her life. She has had no fractures and has lost only ½ inch in height. She began menopause at age 52 and started estrogen replacement for hot flashes. After 1 year of therapy, she stopped and never took estrogen again. Today she has a dietary calcium intake of 800 milligrams a day, and she exercises once or twice a week at her senior center. She was adopted and does not know her family history. Recently, she had a fasting blood cholesterol level of 300, an increase of 80 points since her last cholesterol test 2 years ago.

When Georgia's bone mineral density was measured at the femoral neck of the hip it was 0.60 g/cm^2, and the T score was -2.5.

Georgia has osteoporosis, as defined by a low bone mineral density of the femoral neck in the hip. Even though she has not fractured any bones, her risk of fracturing is very high because her bones are thin. At this time, she needs a medication to prevent her from losing any more bone.

We recommend that Georgia first start to increase her bone mass by increasing her daily calcium intake to 1500 milligrams by adding a supplement of at least 600 milligrams of either calcium carbonate or calcium citrate and also some vitamin D, either by taking two multiple vitamins a day or taking a calcium supplement with added vitamin D. The calcium supplement can cause constipation, so Georgia may need to add some fiber to her diet to prevent this problem.

Georgia also needs to have an antiresorptive agent and a cholesterol-lowering drug added to her medications. It is common for women to increase their cholesterol level as they age. Estrogen keeps the LDL cholesterol low and the HDL cholesterol high.

Georgia should see her doctor a few weeks after she starts taking calcium to make sure that she is tolerating it and that the levels in the blood and urine are safe. Her doctor should also recheck her cholesterol a few months after starting her estrogen treatment to see if it has dropped or if more medication is needed.

About 1 or 2 years after Georgia starts her antiresorptive therapy, her doctor may require another bone mineral density test to determine if the medication is working. There is no exact time that the repeat test should be done. Also, since the medications are very effective, the doctor may decide not to get another bone mineral density test and just to measure her height every year. Georgia will need to know that she will probably have to take this medication for the rest of her life.

7

Medications Other Than Hormones to Prevent and Treat Osteoporosis

Other therapies are now available for the postmenopausal woman who wants to prevent osteoporosis. These include calcitonins, bisphosphonates, vitamin D therapy, and calcium. They have all been studied, and all prevent or decrease bone loss in postmenopausal women. Recent evidence also shows that all of these medications can prevent fractures. These compounds will be discussed in more detail in this chapter.

CALCIUM

Calcium, a mineral, may be the most common prescription given for the treatment of osteoporosis. We know that calcium helps growing bones in young adults achieve their peak mass. We also know that calcium supplements, generally exceeding 1 gram a day, can slow the loss of bone mass in women after menopause, whether or not they have had an osteoporotic fracture. Women who had their ovaries removed and were treated with either a placebo (an inactive tablet) or calcium found that calcium, in a dose of 1 gram a day or more, slowed the rate of bone loss by about 50 percent, especially in cortical bone. For women who are many years postmenopausal, calcium supplements in a dose of at least 1 gram a day can decrease bone loss in both cortical (outer bone) and trabecular (inside bone, next to bone marrow) bone.

Calcium's effect on bone is probably directly related to its effect on bone turnover. As discussed in Chapter 2, with age the calcium balance changes in most adults and less calcium is absorbed. This results in an increase in parathyroid hormone, which draws calcium from the bone and into the bloodstream. Over time, an imbalance in bone turnover is created in which more bone is lost than is formed. The result is a net loss of bone mass. When calcium supplementation is started, parathyroid hormone levels return to normal within a few weeks, bone resorption decreases, and over a year or two, very small increases in bone mass occur. Calcium treatment continues to maintain bone mass for about 3 years; then bone mass may start to decrease slowly again.

Until recently, we did not know whether calcium treatment affected osteoporotic fractures. However, if calcium treatment stopped bone loss, then it was reasonable to assume that it also prevented fractures. A few studies have found that in postmenopausal women who already had osteoporosis and vertebral fractures, and who were treated with calcium supplements and dietary calcium of over 1500 milligrams a day for 2 years, new vertebral fractures decreased.

We also know now that women whose diets are high in calcium and who take high doses of calcium supplements appear to have a decreased risk of hip fractures. Calcium also decreases the risk of hip fractures in women who start taking it even in their late 70s. This is important news because, on average, hip fracture occurs at about age 75 or older. Calcium is highly recommended by all physicians because it is so beneficial and has almost no side effects.

There is another important relationship between calcium and bone: The amount of calcium a child consumes influences the amount and strength of the child's bone mass. When children are growing, the more calcium they get in their diet, the higher the bone mass they will achieve and the stronger their bones will be.

A study was done of college women who were placed at random in either a group that ate a standard diet or a group that ate a standard diet with a calcium supplement. Researchers found that the women who did some regular exercise and added calcium supplements to their diets had more bone growth over a year than those who did not exercise and had a standard diet. Another study of twins added calcium to the diet and studied the effect on bone growth. Each twin group was divided into either a treatment group or a placebo group. The treatment group received a calcium tablet and the placebo group received an identical-looking sugar tablet. At the end of the study, the twins who had received the calcium tablet had a small increase in bone mass compared to the twins who had no added calcium. These studies of college students and twins show that the young skeleton is still growing and will respond to added calcium in the diet, and the addition of calcium will increase bone mass. In light of these findings, it is unfortunate that most Americans take in too little calcium. Most children and adults probably

Table 7.1. *Recommended Daily Amounts of Calcium*

Population Group	Amount (mg/day)
Children and young adults (2 to 24 years)	1200
Men older than 24 years	1000
Women 24 years old to menopause	1000
Women, pregnant or breast-feeding	1600
Women younger than 19 years	1600
Women older than 19 years	1200
Women after menopause	1500
Women not on estrogen but with a risk of osteoporosis	1500
Women on estrogen therapy	1000

consume only about 700 to 800 milligrams a day. A supplement of about 200 to 400 milligrams a day for most adults, young and old, would provide the calcium they need. If the elderly are still eating a balanced diet, this may translate into a supplement of about 700 milligrams a day. If the calcium from dietary sources is low, a higher supplement may be needed.

How Much Calcium Is Needed?

Calcium is needed for all tissues of the body, but especially the bone. The questions that always come up about calcium are: How much calcium should I take? When should I take it, and For how long? The best answer is that we need calcium throughout life, but the optimal amount changes somewhat. The recommended daily amounts, formulated by the National Osteoporosis Foundation, are given in Table 7.1.

Calcium is a nutrient in many foods and should be part of a balanced diet. Examples of foods that are rich in calcium are found in Table 7.2.

If enough calcium is not obtained from food, the next best source is a supplement. Calcium tablets should be taken with meals because food promotes calcium absorption. For most women, a single 200-milligram calcium tablet with one or two meals a day will provide the needed calcium. Calcium tablets come in many doses and sizes. All that you need to remember is that the calcium in the diet and the supplement together should add up to the recommended daily allowance. If young women can take in more calcium both in their diet and with supplements, they will have stronger bones and greater bone

Table 7.2. *Examples of Calcium-Rich Foods*

Food	Serving Size	Milligrams of Calcium	Calories
Fruit yogurt, low fat	1 cup	300	225
Frozen yogurt, low fat	1 cup	200	200
Milk, skim	1 cup	300	90
Pizza, cheese	1 slice	220	290
Salmon, canned, with bones	1 cup	180	120
Cottage cheese, 2%	1 cup	150	200
Beans, dried and cooked	1/2 cup	60–80	115
Tofu (soybean curd)	4 ounces	115	100
Sardines, canned	8 ounces	350	150
Hard cheese	1 ounce	200	100–200
Collard greens, cooked	1 cup	360	100
Bok choy	1 cup	230	80
Broccoli, stalk	1	160–170	70
Orange juice, calcium fortified	1 cup	320	80
Orange	1 medium	60	70

Source: Adapted from Greenwood, S. *Menopause, Naturally* (Updated). Volcano, CA: Volcano Press, 1992.

mass, which will prepare them for later life. For women more than 5 to 7 years past menopause, calcium will slow the rate of bone loss.

Also, it is important to know that if you consume large amounts of cola drinks, caffeinated beverages, and salt, this can increase calcium excretion in your urine, and you will need to increase the calcium in your diet or by supplements to get the daily requirement.

Forms of Calcium Supplements

When you visit your local pharmacy or grocery store to buy calcium supplements, you may be confused by the bewildering array. Here are some tips to help you make the right choices.

Calcium Carbonate
Calcium carbonate is the preferred calcium supplement for young and old alike. It has the highest percentage of calcium per tablet, and it is not very expensive. It has about 40 percent per milligram of calcium, and tablets come in 500- and 650-milligram doses. Usually women take 400 to 2000 milligrams of calcium a day in divided doses. Most people, both young and old, absorb calcium carbonate well. To help absorption, the supplement should be taken with food.

A number of trade names are used to market calcium carbonate; Tums® is one of them.

Calcium Citrate

Another good supplement is calcium citrate, but this has only about 21 percent calcium in each tablet. It may, however, be better than calcium carbonate for people who do not have much stomach acid, as they may absorb it a little better than calcium carbonate. Calcium citrate is more expensive than calcium carbonate. It comes in 950- and 1500-milligram tablets. Remember, most women should supplement their diets with 400 to 500 milligrams of calcium a day, depending on their individual need.

Other Forms of Calcium

Another supplement, calcium gluconate, has only 9 percent calcium and is generally supplied in tablets containing 500 and 600 milligrams. Calcium lactate, still another calcium salt, is 13 percent calcium. The tablets come in 325 and 650 milligrams. Calcium phosphate dibasic, which is 23 percent calcium, is available in 486-milligram tablets. Tricalcium phosphate is 39 percent calcium and comes in 300- and 600-milligram tablets.

Choosing a Calcium Supplement

Here is a general rule for buying a calcium supplement that may be helpful. Calcium tablets tend to be large, and it is important that they dissolve in the gastrointestinal tract so that the calcium can be absorbed. When you buy a calcium supplement, take it home and put one tablet in a glass of very warm (not hot) water. About 10 minutes later, come back and see if the tablet has dissolved at all. If it has, there is a good chance that it will dissolve in your body and allow the calcium to be absorbed. If not, there is a good chance that it will not help you.

Some calcium preparations are combined with vitamin D; one example is OsCal®. This pill contains calcium carbonate and 200 IU of vitamin D. This is a good combination because vitamin D promotes calcium absorption. When you take the two medications together, you may be able to absorb more calcium from each tablet. But it is important to remember that most women can obtain plenty of vitamin D from their diets and from sunlight, so the additional vitamin D in

Table 7.3. *Over-the-Counter Calcium and Vitamin D Preparations*

Brand	Ingredients	Dosage	% Daily Value	Tablets
Nature Made	Calcium carbonate	333 mg	33%	3
OsCal	Calcium carbonate	500 mg	50%	2 or 3
OsCal Calcium + D	Calcium oyster shell,	250 mg	25%	3 or 4
	vitamin D_3	125 IU	31%	
Calcet	Calcium carbonate	150 mg	15%	4
Triplet Calcium+D	Calcium lactate, calcium			
	gluconate, vitamin D_3	400 IU	100%	
One-a-Day "Women's" Multiple	Dicalcium phosphate	500 mg	50%	1 or 2
Vitamin	D-Calcium pantothenate,			
	vitamin D_3	400 IU	100%	
Citracal Calcium	Calcium citrate	400 mg	40%	2 to 4
Citracal Calcium+D	Calcium citrate,	630 mg	63%	1 or 2
	vitamin D_3	400 IU	100%	
Posture Calcium	Tricalcium phosphate	600 mg	60%	1 or 2
Caltrate	Calcium carbonate	600 mg	60%	1 or 2
Calcium + D	Vitamin D_3	200 IU	50%	
Tums 500 Calcium Supplement	Calcium carbonate	500 mg	50%	2 or 3
Geritol Complete Multiple	Dicalcium phosphate	162 mg	16%	1
Vitamin	D-Calcium pantothenate,			
	vitamin D_3	400 IU		
Upjohn Unicap Sr. (for persons	Dicalcium phosphate	100 mg	10%	1 or 2
> 51 years of age)	D-Calcium pantothenate,			
	vitamin D_3	200 IU	50%	
Walgreens Calcium +	Calcium carbonate	500 mg	50%	2
Vitamin D	Vitamin D_2—			
	ergocalciferol	125 IU	35%	

Note: These preparations were randomly selected from a local drug store. In making a choice, review the section on calcium preparations to understand the daily requirements and which calcium preparations are well absorbed.

the OsCal tablet may not be necessary. Furthermore, the combination medication is more expensive than a calcium supplement alone.

Do not forget to tell your physician that you are taking a calcium supplement, as well as the amount. It is important for the doctor to check the amount of calcium in your blood and urine while you are on the supplement to make sure that the level is safe. Common over-the-counter calcium preparations are listed in Table 7.3.

Do You Have Problems Taking Calcium?

Most of the time, calcium supplements cause no problems and are very safe. Some side effects do occur, including bloating, flatulence, or constipation, but these are uncommon. If your calcium supplement causes problems, discuss them with your doctor and possibly switch to another type. Sometimes small changes, like splitting up the dose, crushing the tablet and taking it in orange juice, or putting it in yogurt can help.

Sometimes women who start taking calcium supplements while getting enough calcium from their diet may take in too much calcium and begin excreting it in their urine. If this high calcium intake continues, over time, a painful calcium kidney stone may develop. To protect against this possibility, after you have taken the calcium supplement for 2 to 3 weeks, your doctor should check the calcium in your urine at a laboratory. If it is above normal, a diuretic (a pill to help you excrete water, sometimes known as a *water pill*) can be prescribed to decrease the calcium in the urine, or the amount of calcium taken can be reduced. If a woman has a prior or present history of calcium kidney stones, the calcium in her urine should be checked before the calcium treatment begins. The amount of calcium given in supplement form should be adjusted as necessary.

Also, some women have a disease called *sarcoid* or take large amounts of vitamin D. These women must be careful in taking a calcium supplement because vitamin D increases calcium absorption, and too much vitamin D can result in large concentrations of calcium in the urine, which may lead to problems.

BISPHOSPHONATES

For the Treatment of Osteoporosis

Bisphosphonates (previously called *diphosphonates*) are analogs of the chemical compound pyrophosphate (see Figure 7.1). They have the special property of being absorbed directly by the surface of bone, usually at the sites where active turnover is going on. These compounds also have a special chemical structure that is relatively impervious to degradation. This structure allows these compounds to be absorbed on the surface of bone tissue.

What is special about the bisphosphonates is their ability to prevent bone loss. Bisphosphonates interfere with or inhibit bone resorption by sitting on the bone surface and preventing osteoclast cells, which break down bone, from attaching to the bone or releasing the enzymes that dissolve bone. However, they do not destroy the osteoclasts.

Bisphosphonates reduce the rate at which new bone remodeling

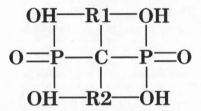

Figure 7.1 *The generic structure of the bisphosphonate compounds. R1 and R2 positions are for side-chains that are unique to each bisphosphonate.*

units are formed. The result is a modest increase (about 1 to 3 percent a year) in bone mass over a few years of treatment, after which a plateau may be reached. Moreover, bisphosphonates decrease bone resorption but allow normal bone formation, so they produce an increase in bone mass or bone balance at each bone remodeling site. A decrease in bone resorption depth protects against loss of trabecular (interior) bone and, as a result, maintains or improves bone quality, reducing the risk of osteoporotic fractures.

Interestingly, oral bisphosphonates are not well absorbed—typically, less than 5 percent. Also, absorption is greatly reduced if the drug is taken with calcium, or with calcium-containing food or beverages, or with just about any food. The bisphosphonate alendronate should be taken on an empty stomach with a glass of water. The person should then remain standing or sitting up for 30 minutes. After that time, the person may eat.

Between 20 and 50 percent of the absorbed drug binds to bone within 12 to 24 hours. Afterward, bone remodeling buries the drug in the bone tissue, where it is retained for months to years but is no longer active. Bisphosphonates are not broken down in the body. The part of the drug that does not bind to the bone sites is excreted in the urine unchanged. Because the drug is eliminated through the kidney, it should be given with caution to patients with kidney problems.

Forms of Bisphosphonate

The First Generation: Etidronate

There are three forms, or generations, of the bisphosphonates (see Table 7.4), and no doubt there will be more in the future. A first-generation bisphosphonate, etidronate, was approved for use in Paget's disease, a condition that results in bone pain because of too much

Table 7.4. *The Three Generations of the Bisphosphonate Compounds*

Generation	Examples
First generation	Etidronate
	Clodronate
Second generation	Alendronate
	Pamidronate
	Tiludronate
	Ibandronate
Third generation	Residronate

remodeling. This medication works by slowing the bone remodeling process. After etidronate was approved and used in Paget's disease, it was studied in women with osteoporosis. Etidronate treatment increased bone mass and reduced new vertebral fractures after 2 years of treatment compared to the placebo group. Unfortunately, in the third year of a three-year study, the differences in vertebral fracture rates between the etidronate and placebo groups were not great, and the Food and Drug Administration did not approve etidronate for the prevention and treatment of osteoporosis.

However, etidronate was already available for the treatment of Paget's disease, so it could be prescribed for osteoporosis. And since, in 1990, there were no medications for the treatment of osteoporosis other than estrogens and injections of calcitonin, physicians started using etidronate to treat osteoporosis.

Etidronate, like all bisphosphonates, is a safe drug. It is taken orally, and very little of the medication—less than 5 percent—is absorbed into the bloodstream. Women who take etidronate for osteoporosis take it for 2 weeks and then stop taking it for the next 11 weeks. This is referred to as *cyclic therapy*. The reason for this schedule is that etidronate inhibits both bone resorption and bone formation if given in high doses continuously. When given for 2 weeks every 3 months, it is safe and effective for the treatment of osteoporosis.

The Second Generation: Alendronate

Recently, a second-generation bisphosphonate, alendronate, has been approved for the treatment and prevention of osteoporosis. Alendronate, unlike first-generation bisphosphonates like etidronate, inhibits bone resorption but has no effect on bone formation. When women with osteoporosis were treated for 3 years, they had about a 6 percent increase in lumbar spine bone mass and a 2 to 4 percent increase in hip bone mass compared to women treated with a placebo. In another study, the Fracture Intervention Study (FIT), women with established osteoporosis (nearly 70 percent had a least one vertebral fracture) were randomized to receive either alendronate or a placebo. After 3 years, bone mineral density at the spine had increased about 5 percent in the women treated with alendronate compared to the placebo group. The most exciting result of this study was that in the women with no vertebral fracture, alendronate decreased the chance of developing a new fracture by nearly 50 percent, and it decreased the risk by 90 percent in women who had had a vertebral fracture at the start of the study. This result clearly establishes alendronate as both a safe and effective therapy for the treatment of established osteoporosis. It also gives women a real alternative to estrogen and calcitonin treatment (discussed next) for osteoporosis.

The bisphosphonates, and especially alendronate, work differently than estrogen to prevent bone loss. Estrogen replacement reduces bone turnover. However, the bisphosphonates prevent osteoclasts from attaching to the bone while allowing bone to form at a normal rate. So, bisphosphonates produce a small but continual increase in bone mass. Not only are they a safe and effective alternative to estrogen treatment for osteoporosis, they are probably somewhat more potent antiresorptive agents. It is possible that the combination of bisphosphonates with either estrogen or calcitonin will be even better than any of the medications alone.

The dose of alendronate used for the treatment of osteoporosis is 10 milligrams a day. The only side effect is upper gastrointestinal irritation or esophagitis. To prevent this, as noted earlier, women who take alendronate should take it in the morning, with a glass of warm water. Afterward, they should stand or sit up, eating nothing for 30 minutes. Also, it is important not to cut the tablet in half; doing so changes the protective covering around the medication and increases the risk of gastrointestinal irritation.

The Third Generation

At this time, other bisphosphonates are under development and will soon be approved for the treatment and prevention of osteoporosis. These new medications include residronate and ibandronate. Some of them are given by tablets and others by injection. They all appear to be safe and may have fewer gastrointestinal problems than the bisphosphonates that are currently approved. The bisphosphonate compounds are a real breakthrough for the treatment of osteoporosis, and the next set of bisphosphonate medications should be even better.

For the Prevention of Osteoporosis

Recently, alendronate has been approved for the prevention of osteoporosis. Prevention means that a woman can take a medication before she has the disease. Alendronate, at a dose of 5 milligrams a day, was tested in women who were within 1 to 3 years of menopause. At the end of the 2-year study, women treated with alendronate and estrogen maintained their bone mass, while those treated with a placebo had a small (1 to 2 percent) loss of bone mass. At the end of the 5-year study, women treated with either alendronate or estrogen also continued to maintain their bone mass, while those treated with the placebo lost bone mass. Therefore, alendronate at a dose of 5 milligrams a day is as effective as estrogen to prevent bone loss in women early in menopause. However, it should not be a first-line agent for the prevention of osteoporosis. Remember, the number one cause of death among women is heart disease, and estrogen reduces this risk by nearly 40 percent. Estrogen also prevents hot flashes, vaginal dryness, dementia, skin wrinkling, and osteoporosis. So, while alendronate is as effective as estrogen in preventing bone loss and osteoporosis, the many other health benefits of estrogen still make it the treatment of choice.

Who Should Take Bisphosphonates Instead of HRT for Prevention of Osteoporosis

If a woman definitely cannot take estrogen because she has a personal history of breast cancer or two first-degree relatives with breast cancer, or because she cannot tolerate estrogen and has either low bone mass or a strong family history of osteoporosis, then alendronate is the appropriate medication for her.

Another important question is, who should take alendronate for the prevention of osteoporosis? Since the only benefit of alendronate is to prevent bone loss, a woman should not take it unless she has low bone density. For a woman who is starting menopause and is not planning to take estrogen, the best thing is to have a bone mineral density test. This test will indicate her risk of osteoporosis. If her bone mineral density is normal, she does not need to prevent bone loss. Instead, she should exercise, establish good health and dietary habits, and have a repeat bone mass measurement in about 2–5 years. If she then has low bone mineral density, she may want to start alendronate or calcitonin therapy to prevent further bone loss.

CALCITONIN

Calcitonin is a hormone that circulates in the body. It is produced by the thyroid gland in addition to thyroid hormones. Calcitonin acts on the bone by decreasing osteoclastic bone resorption, which stops bone loss.

Calcitonin has been approved by the Food and Drug Administration for the treatment of postmenopausal osteoporosis. At first, calcitonin was available only as an injection under the skin. Recently, however, the Food and Drug Administration approved the use of a nasal spray. This new preparation makes the medication much easier to use.

Benefits

Since calcitonin, like estrogen and the bisphosphonates, blocks bone resorption, it maintains bone or prevents bone loss in women who are estrogen deficient at the beginning of menopause; it also prevents bone loss in women who have established osteoporosis. Calcitonin has the most dramatic effects in women with high bone turnover. This condition occurs with early estrogen deficiency at menopause. It also may occur in the later years of menopause and in bone diseases other other than osteoporosis.

Calcitonin preserves bone mass and prevents fractures. When women who were within 3 years of starting menopause were treated with calcitonin for 2 years, calcitonin preserved their vertebral bone mass, while women treated with a placebo lost bone mass. Other studies using both subcutaneous (injected just under the skin) and intranasal preparations have found that in early menopause, calcitonin prevents bone loss both in the vertebral bone and in the cortical bone of the forearm. (Calcitonin is not currently approved by the Food and Drug Administration in the United States for prevention of osteoporosis.)

Calcitonin has also been used to prevent bone loss and new fractures in women with established osteoporosis. Women with osteoporotic fractures who were treated with calcitonin gained bone mass in both the vertebrae and the forearm during the 1 year of treatment. They also experienced a decrease in fractures. In a study of over 5000 men and women 50 years of age or older, involving subjects from six countries in southern Europe, researchers demonstrated that calcitonin, like estrogen, significantly decreased the development of hip fractures. Calcitonin therapy for 2 years also greatly reduced vertebral fracture rates in osteoporotic women 15 to 22 years after menopause, who had entered the study with at least one vertebral fractures. In fact, when calcitonin was administered by nasal spray to postmenopausal women for 2 years, the incidence of new fractures was reduced by over 50 percent—even though the change in bone mass in the lumbar spine in the calcitonin-treated group was only about 2 percent different from the placebo-treated group.

Calcitonin, like estrogen and the bisphosphonates, must be used indefinitely to preserve bone mass in women with established osteoporosis or to prevent osteoporosis. The usual dose of nasal calcitonin is 200 IU a day. The form of calcitonin given by injection is salmon calcitonin (Calcimar® or Miacalcin®) subcutaneously or intramuscularly (into the muscle) in a dose of 50 to 100 IU.

Side Effects

Some women treated with calcitonin develop nausea or mild gastrointestinal discomfort. These symptoms usually occur at the beginning of the treatment but then typically disappear. Some women complain of facial flushing and of itchiness in the areas where the injections are given. The itching also tends to disappear. If it continues, a mild antihistamine can be taken about 30 minutes before the subcutaneous injection of calcitonin is given. Side effects tend to be greater when the medication is given subcutaneously than when it is given by a nasal spray.

Relief of Pain

A unique and unexpected finding is that calcitonin is a potent pain reliever. Osteoporotic patients with a vertebral fracture often have severe pain. The strong pain medications derived from morphine, like codeine, Percodan®, or Vicodin®, relieve the pain but frequently cause constipation, and the strain of having a bowel movement can make the back pain worse. Calcitonin works without causing constipation and relieves pain, which is very welcome to patients with an acute vertebral fracture. Osteoporotic patients with pain generally are treated with either 200 IU per day of a nasal spray or 100 IU per day of a subcutaneous injection 5 to 7 days a week. After 2 to 4 weeks, the pain from the new fracture should be relieved. The medication can be reduced and eventually stopped altogether. If calcitonin is used to treat osteoporosis, the dose should remain at either 200 IU per day of the nasal spray or 100 IU per day of the subcutaneous injection indefinitely.

DECIDING WHICH THERAPY TO CHOOSE

With the many types of medication now available to treat osteoporosis, patients and physicians need to discuss the best options. In general, all women should be started on HRT because of its beneficial cardiovascular effects and the protection it provides against osteoporosis. But some women may not be able to start HRT, perhaps because of a history of breast cancer or migraine headaches or because of personal objections. Calcitonin is an appropriate medication for women who, for one reason or another, cannot or do not choose to take estrogen. Calcitonin, when used early in menopause, prevents bone loss and future fractures. Its use in later menopause or with established osteoporosis also prevents new vertebral fractures and other nonvertebral fractures. A woman with postmenopausal osteoporosis who will not take estrogen or a bisphosphonate should take calcitonin; any medication that will prevent bone loss is better than no medication at all. Also, with the new nasal formula, more women may be willing to take it.

Another benefit of calcitonin is that even though it is potent, it is essentially without side effects, especially compared to other medications used to treat osteoporosis. This is important because elderly postmenopausal women may be taking several medications to manage other diseases. At this time, although I do not recommend calcitonin as a first-line agent for the prevention and treatment of osteoporosis, it is an effective anti–bone-resorbing agent and can be used as an alternative to estrogen. It prevents bone loss with estrogen deficiency, and with established osteoporosis it prevents new fractures. As a natural hormone that is already in the body, calcitonin is generally safe. Its availability as a nasal spray has also made it easier to use.

WHEN IS A BISPHOSPHONATE PREFERABLE TO CALCITONIN?

In general, the bisphosphonates are more potent than calcitonin in preventing bone loss. Calcitonin prevents bone loss and maintains the bone mass at about the same level. Calcitonin's major effect is in the spine. The bisphosphonates prevent further bone loss and actually increase bone mass a small percentage every year. Therefore, if a woman must use a medication to prevent bone loss, either a bisphosphonate or calcitonin will be effective. A woman can then decide if she wants to take a tablet (bisphosphonate) or use a nasal spray (calcitonin). If a woman has low bone mass or osteoporosis and has had a bone fracture, a bisphosphonate is preferable to calcitonin because the bisphosphonate will increase her bone mass a little every year and decrease the risk of another fracture. Calcitonin will prevent her from losing more bone but probably will not increase bone mass, and it is less effective in preventing another fracture. However, if a woman is unable to take a bisphosphonate, calcitonin is a very good alternative.

WHEN IS A BISPHOSPHONATE OR CALCITONIN MORE OR LESS EFFECTIVE THAN HRT?

In general, when a woman wants a medication to prevent bone loss, bisphosphonates, HRT, and calcitonin are all equally effective. The decision depends on whether the woman wants to prevent other diseases. If a woman in early menopause wants to prevent bone loss, and there is no history of breast cancer in her first-degree relatives, she should take HRT. However, if there is a family history of breast cancer or if the woman does not want to take HRT and has low bone mass, she should take either a bisphosphonate or calcitonin.

In a woman who has osteoporosis and low bone mass, HRT, bisphosphonates, and, to a lesser extent, calcitonin will prevent new fractures and increase bone mass. Again, the woman must decide. If she will not take HRT, the bisphosphonates or calcitonin will be effective in preventing fractures and improving bone mass. If a woman with osteoporosis is unable to take bisphosphonates, calcitonin is a good alternative.

Today, women are lucky because they have choices among medications to treat osteoporosis. It is important for a woman to discuss her concerns with her doctor to understand the benefits and risks of each medication.

SUMMARY

- Other therapies are available for postmenopausal women who want to prevent or treat osteoporosis.

- Calcium and vitamin D, both in food and in supplements, help maintain bone mass and are essential for bone health.
- The bisphosphonates and calcitonin stop or slow bone breakdown. They prevent bone loss and actually increase bone mass modestly in osteoporotic women and men.
- A bisphosphonate or calcitonin should be taken to prevent osteoporosis by a woman who cannot take estrogen (due to a personal or family history of cancer), who cannot tolerate estrogen, and who has either low bone mass or a strong family history of osteoporosis.

PATRICIA: PREVENTING OSTEOPOROSIS IN MIDDLE AGE

Patricia, a 38-year-old woman, is 5 feet 7 inches tall and weighs about 125 pounds. She had two full-term pregnancies and now has two teenage children. She has a family history of osteoporosis. Her mother fell and suffered a hip fracture at age 71, and her paternal grandmother had compression fractures of the spine in her 70s. Patricia eats a normal diet, and her calcium intake each day, which she gets from two or three glasses of milk, a serving of frozen yogurt, and vegetables, is about 700 milligrams. She exercises three times a week by running for about 30 minutes and has never broken a bone. She has had normal menstrual periods since she began menstruating at around age 14.

Recently, Patricia had a bone mineral density measurement of her lumbar spine. Her bone density was 0.92 g/cm^2, which is normal for her age. Her T score was 0.091, which is also normal. In spite of a family history of osteoporosis, she has normal bone mass as she enters middle age. The factors that have probably helped her achieve normal bone mass are her normal age of menarche and her regular weight-bearing exercise.

Patricia has a very good chance of preventing osteoporosis because of her normal peak bone mass. She would have to lose a great deal of bone before she risks developing an osteoporotic fracture. But it is important to remember that Patricia is only 38 years old and that the symptoms of osteoporosis do not generally develop until the mid-70s. Patricia will need to prevent bone loss by maintaining her exercise and healthy diet.

Patricia should continue her regular weight-bearing exercise, which helps to maintain her present bone mass. But she must increase her calcium intake to over 1000 milligrams a day and add vitamin D, in the form of a multiple vitamin, to ensure that she absorbs as much calcium as possible. She can increase her calcium intake to normal by adding just one calcium carbonate or calcium gluconate supplement. These changes will probably work for Patricia until she undergoes menopause.

Patricia will probably not go through menopause until the age of 50. When menopause begins, it would be prudent for her to obtain another bone mineral density test of her spine or hip to determine her bone mass and her risk of developing an osteoporotic fracture at that time. She should also definitely consider taking a medication to prevent bone loss because she has a strong family history of osteoporosis. She will also need to increase her calcium supplement to 1500 milligrams a day.

MARION: A PREMENOPAUSAL WOMAN WITH HABITS THAT PUT HER AT RISK OF DEVELOPING OSTEOPOROSIS

Marion is a 45-year-old woman, 5 feet 4 inches tall, who weighs about 110 pounds. She has had five children and has used birth control pills for 20 years. Her mother died when she was young, and she does not know the history of osteoporosis on her mother's side of the family. Her paternal grandmother had a hip fracture at the age of 85. Marion has smoked cigarettes for 30 years, generally about one pack a day. She also drinks five or six cups of coffee a day and two or three large glasses of wine each night. Her calcium intake is 500 to 600 milligrams a day, and she takes one multiple vitamin a day that provides about 400 IU of vitamin D.

When Marion's bone mineral density was measured in her spine, the reading was 0.75 g/cm^2 and her T score was -1.5, which is below normal for her age. The reason is most likely a combination of factors—genetics, low calcium intake, and a long history of smoking.

The nicotine in cigarettes does a number of things to bone. First, it increases estrogen breakdown, which over a long period of time can result in low bone mass. Nicotine also decreases the population of cells that form bone, which results in low bone mass. Heavy smokers also tend to go through menopause earlier, so their bodies have low estrogen levels for more years. Given all these facts, to prevent further bone loss, Marion should quit smoking. Although she has smoked for a long time, there are very good programs that can help her. The sooner she gets the nicotine out of her body, the better off she will be. First, the estrogen she already produces will remain in the bloodstream longer. Second, since she is premenopausal, she may not go through early menopause, which would, of course, lower her estrogen level indefinitely.

Marion should also increase her calcium intake to about 1200 milligrams a day. She can do this by increasing the calcium in her diet and by taking a supplement of either calcium carbonate or another preparation.

She should also try to decrease her alcohol intake to one glass of wine or one cocktail a day. Although Marion is not a heavy drinker, women who drink alcohol tend to let alcohol replace their usual diets and fail to get all the nutrients they need from a normal diet. But more important, alcohol suppresses bone formation, so a modest intake is best.

Finally, Marion should continue her usual exercise class since the exercise may have prevented the loss of more bone mass than was caused by her smoking.

FRANCES: ALTERNATIVES TO ESTROGEN—BISPHOSPHONATES OR CALCITONIN FOR THE TREATMENT OF POSTMENOPAUSAL OSTEOPOROSIS

Frances is a 55-year-old brown-haired woman with fair skin. She is 5 feet 1 inch tall and weighs 95 pounds. Her menopause began at age 50, and currently she has hot flashes at least once a day. Over the past 10 years, prior to menopause, she noticed that her menstrual periods lasted only 3 days and the bleeding was light. She has no children and used birth control pills for about 5 years from age 25 to 30. Her mother had breast cancer at age 45 and died of the disease at age 50. Her sister is 57 and had breast cancer diagnosed 1 year ago.

Frances smoked one pack of cigarettes a day for 10 years, from age 30 to 40, and she drinks about one glass of wine a day. She has been an exercise fanatic for 15 years. She runs 50 miles each week and competes in long-distance races, usually in marathons, twice a year. She uses no medications on a regular basis.

Her daily calcium intake through diet and a daily multiple vitamin is about 900 milligrams, and her vitamin D intake is about 800 IU a day.

When Frances's bone mineral density was measured in her lumbar spine, her reading was 0.78 and her T score was −2.0—low for her age.

We do not know all the reasons, but she is small-boned and thin. She is also a serious runner, and the change in her menstrual periods that accompanied her increase in exercise may have resulted in low circulating estrogen levels and further bone loss. At any rate, she has now gone through menopause and has a low bone mass. If she loses more bone, she will have an increased risk of an osteoporotic fracture. Frances needs a medication to prevent further bone loss. The usual first step would be estrogen therapy, but with a family history of breast cancer in two first-degree relatives, this is not recommended. Luckily the last few years have brought more medications to treat and prevent osteoporosis, so Frances has options.

Treatment can begin with either a bisphosphonate or calcitonin, both of which will prevent further bone loss. Frances will also need to increase her calcium intake to 1500 milligrams a day. This can be done by taking a calcium supplement that provides 600 milligrams. The rest of her calcium should come from food. Frances should also have her height measured in her doctor's office. Height changes are a very simple way for a doctor to determine if a patient has developed vertebral fractures. With these fractures, individuals can lose several inches of height. After about a year, Frances should have her bone mineral density measured again to see if her medication is preventing further bone loss. If she has lost more than 5 percent of the bone mineral density in her lumbar spine in the first year of treatment, her doctor should consider adding another medication to prevent further bone loss. The doctor may also want to order biochemical tests to measure her rate of bone remodeling.

Another option for Frances to consider is a medication that may prevent breast cancer and bone loss at the same time. Tamoxifen has been used for many years to treat women with advanced breast cancer. These patients who were treated with tamoxifen for many years did not lose bone mass. This is probably because tamoxifen was acting like an antiestrogen in the breast tissue but like estrogen in the bone. A large national study is now being done to treat women with a strong family history of breast cancer with tamoxifen to see if it can prevent this cancer. These women are also having their bone mineral density measured. We will soon know the answer to this important question.

Tamoxifen is relatively safe and could be given immediately. Also, raloxifene, another medication like tamoxifen, is now approved for the prevention of osteoporosis. So, in the not too distant future, Frances will have even more options for preventing osteoporosis.

Because Frances is a serious athlete, overexercise and low body weight may result in further bone loss. There has been very little research on this topic so far, but many more middle-aged and elderly women and men now are now committed athletes, and the contribution of intense exercise to bone mass may be another consideration in treating osteoporosis. At this time, the only advice a doctor can give is to maintain weight and not try to lose weight. Weight has a positive effect on bone mass. Also, Frances's bone mass should be checked every few years. If she continues to lose bone mass while exercising intensely despite taking medications to prevent bone loss, then a modified exercise program may be critical. Currently, we do not know enough to make strong recommendations on how much exercise is healthy for middle-aged and elderly individuals.

JANE: THE MEDICATIONS A POSTMENOPAUSAL WOMAN CAN TAKE TO PREVENT OSTEOPOROSIS WHEN SHE MUST STOP USING ESTROGEN

Jane is a 55-year-old white woman, 5 feet 2 inches tall, weighing 125 pounds. She has three children and a strong family history of osteoporosis; both her mother and her father's mother have the disease. Jane began menopause at age 50 and experienced hot flashes and vaginal dryness. A bone mineral density scan of her lumbar spine was slightly below normal. She began to take daily estrogen and progestin therapy. Her physician also had her increase her calcium intake to 1500 milligrams a day and her vitamin D intake to 800 IU a day. After 2 years of hormone therapy, she had a mammogram and a uterine biopsy; both tests were normal.

After 5 years of estrogen therapy, her mammogram showed a possible breast mass. A biopsy was positive for a very early stage of cancer. The cancer was limited to the small mass, and it was removed. Jane had a short course of radiation therapy.

This is a difficult case because the fear of breast cancer is real. Jane developed a breast mass that, by tissue diagnosis, was considered an early breast cancer. But it is important to keep in mind that this mass could have occurred by chance alone or may indeed be related to the 5 years of estrogen therapy. We simply do not know. Either way, Jane should stop her estrogen therapy and use another medication to prevent bone loss. Since Jane has taken estrogen for 5 years, if she stops using it and does not use another medication to prevent bone loss, she will lose whatever bone mass she gained by taking estrogen. Several studies have focused on women who took estrogen for many years and then stopped. They seem to suggest that a woman needs to take estrogen for about 10 years after menopause to obtain maximum protection from osteoporotic fractures. Since Jane has taken estrogen for only 5 years, she should start using another medication to prevent osteoporosis.

This case has an important message for all of us: Regular mammograms while taking estrogen therapy are essential. They can usually detect breast cancers long before they are found by the doctor or patient. If you are considering estrogen therapy, you must be vigilant and take regular mammograms so that if you develop a breast cancer, it can be treated early and successfully.

Since it has been 5 years since Jane had a bone mineral density scan, this would be a good time to repeat it. Initially, Jane had normal bone mineral density for her age and started estrogen therapy to treat her hot flashes. If her repeat bone mineral density scan is again normal, she may not need an antiresorptive bone agent. She can continue to take her daily calcium and vitamin D and have another bone density test in about 2 years. Alternatively, if she has lost bone mass since her initial bone density measurement, her doctor may recommend another antiresorptive agent—either a bisphosphonate like alendronate, calcitonin nasal spray, or raloxifene (a selective estrogen receptor modulator, SERM).

HELEN: A CASE OF ESTABLISHED OSTEOPOROSIS

Helen is a 75-year-old white woman who went through menopause over 25 years ago. She has osteoporosis and has suffered three vertebral fractures, which have reduced her height from 5 feet 3 inches to about 5 feet. When Helen was counseled about osteoporosis about 20 years ago, the only indication that she might be at risk for this disease was that her mother had a hip fracture at the age of 70. Estrogen therapy was recommended at the time of menopause, but she decided against it. Helen also suffers from gastric reflux, for which she takes two Tums tablets three times a day. Her diet is normal, and her only activity is daily housework.

When Helen's bone density was measured at the femoral neck of the hip, it was found to be 0.57 g/cm^2, and her T score was -3.0.

Helen's osteoporosis and compression fractures are probably the result of inheriting low peak bone mass and 25 years of estrogen deficiency since menopause. Her fractures have caused her loss of height and current back pain. In addition, a hump (thoracic kyphosis), has developed in her midback, so that her posture is hunched and her clothes fit oddly.

The bone mineral density test was done at her hip instead of her spine for a number of reasons. First, in a woman over the age of 65, there are changes in the bones of the spine from arthritis and degenerative disc disease, as well as calcifications in the major arteries of the body that pass by the spine. These changes make a lumbar spine scan difficult to interpret. Also, when a woman has suffered osteoporotic fractures, vertebral compression makes interpretation of the bone mineral density tests difficult. Finally, with compression fractures of the spine, it becomes very difficult for a woman to lay flat on her back. For all of these reasons, a bone mineral density scan of the lumbar spine can be difficult to interpert.

Therefore, once a woman is over the age of 65, it is more reliable, and easier for the patient, to obtain a bone mineral density scan of the hip. Luckily, there are many similarities in the bone mass measured at different sites in the body. So, if a bone mineral density scan of the hip is normal, there is a reasonably good chance that the spine will also be normal.

Since Helen has established osteoporosis, it is critical for her to begin medication immediately. She has already fractured three vertebrae, and the bone mineral density in her hip is very low. Any further bone loss will be very serious.

First, Helen needs to increase her calcium intake to 1500 milligrams a day, by adding a supplement of either calcium carbonate or calcium citrate, and to increase her vitamin D intake to 800 IU a day with two multiple vitamins. The calcium and vitamin D will help her maintain her bone mass, especially in the hip or the cortical bone. But this alone is not enough in a woman of her age who has had three vertebral fractures. Helen will also need to take an antiresorptive agent that will prevent her from losing more bone mass. She can take either a bisphosphonate like alendronate, calcitonin nasal spray, or estrogen replacement. All of these medications work about the same way to prevent bone loss and prevent new fractures, so the choice must be based on other aspects of Helen's health and her personal preferences. For example, Helen and her doctor need to assess the risks and benefits of each medication. For example, estrogen replacement therapy will prevent bone loss, and the medication can be taken as either a patch or a tablet. Estrogen would be a good medication to use if Helen has a family history of heart disease because estrogen also prevents heart disease in women. On the other hand, if Helen's uterus is intact, she will have to take progesterone—either a few days a month or a small dose every day to protect against uterine cancer. If she takes the progesterone a few days a month or a few days every 2 to 3 months, she will experience menstrual periods again, and she may not like that. Estrogen use prevents vaginal dryness, and research indicates that it may prevent dementia in women. But it may also increase her risk of developing breast cancer, so every year or two she will need to have a mammogram. The benefits of estrogen must be weighed against the risk in a woman of Helen's age, and the decision must be hers.

Another medication that will prevent Helen from losing bone mass is alendronate, a bisphosphonate. Long-term studies show that alendronate will increase Helen's bone mass 2 to 3 percent over the next 3 to 5 years while decreasing her risk of new vertebral and hip fractures. However, several things need to be kept in mind. Alendronate must be taken first thing in the morning with a glass of water; nothing can be eaten for the next 30 minutes to allow the medication to be absorbed. Occasionally, alendronate causes irritation of the stomach and esophagus; if this occurs, Helen should tell her doctor.

If Helen decides not to take estrogen or alendronate, she could take calcitonin daily in a nasal spray. Calcitonin has very few side effects other than some irritation of the nostrils where the spray touches the membranes of the nose. There is good evidence that calcitonin prevents bone loss in a woman like Helen, but in studies it did not prevent new fractures as well as estrogen and alendronate. This may be partly because these studies were smaller and briefer than those with the other medications. In all likelihood, calcitonin can prevent new fractures about as well as estrogen and alendronate.

At this point, Helen is taking calcium, vitamin D, and an antiresorptive agent. But medications alone are not enough. Helen also needs to see a physical therapist or to enroll in a special exercise class. Compression fractures have created her kyphosis, and she will need help in preventing further injury. Helen has trouble with balance and feels as if she will fall forward at any time. It is also hard for her to move her neck to the side because of her poor posture. In this class, Helen will need to learn back extension exercises that will improve her posture and prevent her from bending forward. The class will also help Helen learn how to move around safely in her home and do household chores like vacuuming and dusting without feeling that she will fall over. The exercises can improve her muscle strength, and with this her balance should improve. In fact, this rehabilitation is the most important part of Helen's treatment. With the many changes her body has undergone, Helen will undoubtedly be concerned about her appearance, as well as with preventing fractures in the future. Her clothes will need to be altered because the vertebral fractures have reduced her height and a forward curve has developed in her back. Her dresses are too long, and her breast size may have increased. And, perhaps most important, Helen's changed appearance and her feeling of poor balance may have reduced her self-esteem. She is probably getting out less often socially. Her doctor and her physical therapist must try to keep Helen connected to her social network because isolation at her age can lead to depression and premature death. Her friends and family must encourage her to go out and must arrange transportation for her if she is not able to travel alone.

What happens next? We often tell patients like Helen many things—what to do as a result of the osteoporosis and fractures—but medication is not the end of the treatment. Helen should see her doctor about her osteoporosis within a few weeks of starting her new medications and after her exercise program is underway. Helen has increased her daily calcium intake, and her doctor must perform blood and urine tests to determine if the new calcium level is safe and appropriate. The doctor must also find out if she is tolerating her new medications. Sometimes the increase in calcium to 1500 milligrams a day can cause constipation. If this occurs, Helen needs to add more fiber to her diet; taking a few tablespoons a day of Metamucil® (a bulk-forming agent) to help produce normal bowel movements will definitely help. If Helen begins to use alendronate, she will be asked if it has caused any gastrointestinal discomfort. If all is well after a follow-up visit, Helen should return in about a year so that the osteoporosis therapy can be appraised and another bone density measurement done.

What happens 12 months later? Helen returns to see her doctor about her osteoporosis. At that time, the doctor should measure her height carefully to see if it has changed over the past year. A new bone mineral density scan will indicate whether the medications have been successful and whether Helen's bone mass is now stable. Luckily, the new bone scan of her hip revealed a 3 percent increase in bone mass over the past year, and Helen's height has not changed. Therefore, Helen should stay on her current medications and return in another year for a repeat evaluation.

Another outcome of the 1-year visit could have been that Helen suffered a new vertebral fracture, identified by a spine X-ray. The bone mineral density of her hip decreased by 7 percent. A new fracture or a decrease in bone mass of more than 7 percent means that her medication is not working. Her doctor could decide to add another antiresorptive medication. If Helen had started using estrogen replacement therapy, her doctor may add alendronate or calcitonin. If she had started using alendronate (10 milligrams a day), her doctor may add estrogen replacement or calcitonin. Very early results from recent studies show that two antiresorptive agents are more effective than either one alone in preventing bone loss. If Helen is started on another antiresorptive agent, she will again return in 1 year, when another bone mineral density scan will be done to determine how the two medications are working together.

MARTHA: ADDING CALCIUM TO THE DIET
OF AN OLDER ADULT

Martha is a 79-year-old Asian woman who is 5 feet tall and weighs 110 pounds. She started menopause at the age of 52 and took estrogen for 13 years, stopping it about 15 years ago because she thought it was no longer helpful. She has no family history of osteoporosis. Her calcium intake is 1000 milligrams a day with her diet and one calcium carbonate supplement. She also takes a multiple vitamin each morning. She walks her dog in a park for 45 minutes each day and volunteers to read to children at the local library. When her bone mineral density was tested at her hip, it was found to be 0.57 g/cm^2, and her T score was -3.0.

Martha, although very thin all of her life, obtained a high peak bone mass. Estrogen replacement therapy for 10 years also ensured that she maintains good bone mass, and her current bone mass is considered low normal. She has a very low risk of fracturing at this time. Martha only needs to maximize her intake of calcium because as women reach the age of 80, their ability to absorb calcium markedly decreases and they lose bone. The bone loss with aging is very different from the bone loss that occurs with menopause, which results from estrogen deficiency. The bone loss that comes with age results partly in slowed bone formation. At the same time, bone resorption is slightly increased because as less calcium is absorbed, parathyroid hormone releases calcium from the bone, resulting in bone loss. The addition of both calcium and vitamin D to the diet of elderly persons stops increased bone resorption and stimulates bone formation. Studies of women in their mid-80s have found that calcium and vitamin D alone preserve bone mass and decrease hip fractures.

The challenge at this point is to find the right calcium for an elderly woman to take. Calcium supplements often cause constipation, which is already a problem in many elderly women. Also, to be absorbed, calcium requires stomach acid. As we age, much less acid is produced, decreasing calcium absorption.

At this point, the only treatment Martha needs is an increase in her calcium intake to 1500 milligrams a day, and for this she needs an additional 500-milligram supplement. Although most calcium preparations are adequate and tolerated, in elderly women I prefer to use calcium citrate. This form of calcium does not need stomach acid to be absorbed, so more of it is absorbed compared to calcium carbonate. If Martha develops constipation with the increase in her daily calcium supplement, I would recommend that she add some fiber to her diet with a few tablespoons of Metamucil® each day. But since Metamucil® may inhibit calcium absorption, the two medications must be taken at different times each day. Luckily, calcium citrate can be purchased over the counter at most drug stores and grocery stores, and the cost is reasonable. Vitamin D is now being formulated in tablets that contain either calcium carbonate or other calcium preparations. These make it easier to remember that vitamin D promotes calcium absorption and should be added whenever calcium needs to be increased in the diet.

JOHN: A MAN WHO FRACTURED HIS HIP

John is an 82-year-old man who fractured his left hip. He was in good health all of his life and retired at age 65 from his job as an accountant. His mother had osteoporosis and fractured her hip at the age of 75, and his sister, who is 85 years old, has several vertebral compression fractures. John is currently 5 feet 9 inches tall and weighs 150 pounds. His usual calcium intake is about 700 milligrams a day, and he walks about five blocks a day for exercise.

Most men who develop osteoporosis suffer hip fractures, which usually do not happen until after the age of 80. Because men start out with more bone mass than women and do not go through menopause, their testosterone level does not change, as the estrogen level does with women at menopause. So bone loss from sex hormone deficiency does not occur in men. But men, like women, do experience age-related bone loss. As men age, they absorb less calcium and their bone resorption increases. With age, bone formation is also reduced, so that men lose up to 1 to 2 percent of bone mass every year after about the age of 70. Therefore, men who have low bone mass and who lose an additional 10-20 percent from the age of 75 to 85 are at very high risk of having an osteoporotic fracture.

John has a family history of osteoporosis, and he inherited a small frame and low bone mass. In addition, with age, he lost more bone mass and eventually suffered a hip fracture.

Unfortunately, there are no good studies on the treatment of osteoporosis in men. However, we know enough about the abnormalities in the bone turnover cycle to make reasonable recommendations for John. Adequate calcium and vitamin D intake will prevent John from losing any more bone mass. Therefore, he needs to increase his calcium intake from 700 to 1500 milligrams a day by adding a supplement, and 800 IU of vitamin D a day either by taking two daily multiple vitamins or by taking a calcium supplement that also contains vitamin D, such as OsCal or Citrical+ D. Also, at this time, John's testosterone level should be checked to determine if part of his bone loss is from testosterone deficiency. If his testosterone level is low, he and his doctor can discuss treatment with testosterone. Testosterone acts like an antiresorptive agent for bone and may also increase bone formation. If John's testosterone level is normal, he and his doctor may decide that he should use another antiresorptive agent, either a bisphosphonate or calcitonin intranasal spray.

Also, after hip surgery, John may have trouble walking, as his balance and his stride may be different than they were before the hip fracture and surgery. It is important that John see a physical therapist after surgery to determine if he might benefit from a cane or another device to promote good balance. He should also be evaluated for other potential risk factors for hip fractures that could be corrected. For example, he needs to visit his eye doctor to make sure that his depth perception is is normal; if it is not, he will need a prescription for eyeglasses. Also, since a sedentary lifestyle increases the risk of a hip fracture, John should join an exercise class that meets a few times a week for low-impact exercises to improve his strength and balance and prevent another fall. Lastly, a visiting nurse or therapist should come to his home to see if there are any places where he might easily fall—for example, a step without a side rail or a cracked tile that could catch his foot and cause him to lose his balance. Making the home of an older person fall-proof is the most important thing that can be done to prevent future falls.

8
The Role of Vitamin D

BONE DISEASES FROM VITAMIN D DEFICIENCY

There are many theories about the effect of vitamins on bone. The one vitamin that is most closely connected with bone is vitamin D. Vitamin D's target tissue is bone. A childhood disease resulting from vitamin D deficiency is *rickets*; in adults, the resulting disease is called *osteomalacia*. With vitamin D deficiency, bone tissue fails to mineralize or become hard and stiff. In children with rickets, growth areas of the bone do not mineralize. Luckily, unless there is a genetic syndrome that prevents vitamin D from working, both rickets and osteomalacia are readily cured by vitamin D replacement. Vitamin D is probably the best studied of all the naturally occurring vitamins. Yet, despite decades of research, many questions about its role in bone metabolism remain, and we are not certain about how it acts directly on bones.

Osteoporosis is the end product of a complicated process leading to a reduction of bone mass to the point where fractures occur with very little stress. Many conditions lead to osteoporosis, including sex hormone deficiency, steroid use, thyroid or parathyroid hormone excess, calcium deficiency, and immobilization. Unlike the well-established role of vitamin D in the treatment or prevention of rickets or osteomalacia, its role in the management of osteoporosis is much less certain.

THE ROLE OF VITAMIN D IN
MAINTAINING HEALTHY BONE

Vitamin D in its active form—1,25 dihydroxyvitamin D—promotes bone turnover. This form of vitamin D promotes maturation of both osteoclast and osteoblast cells. Its effect on bone turnover overall is not known.

Vitamin D enhances bone metabolism by promoting intestinal calcium absorption. Calcium deficiency leads to a decrease in bone mass, and adequate calcium is needed to attain peak bone mass. At the other end of life, when osteoporosis may be present several questions arise. For example, can a fall in calcium intake or intestinal calcium absorption be responsible, at least in part, for the accelerated bone loss at menopause or the gradual loss of bone with aging? Because 1,25 dihydroxyvitamin D is the main regulator of intestinal calcium absorption, are there any changes in the level of this vitamin, or tissue resistance to it, that may cause the change in calcium absorption with menopause or aging? The known answers will now be discussed.

Calcium Levels in Older Women

Most studies show that intestinal calcium absorption declines with age, especially in women who are osteoporotic. Also, as we age, the amount of dietary calcium we need to maintain our bodily calcium balance increases. Postmenopausal women treated with vitamin D increase their intestinal calcium absorption. Estrogen treatment of postmenopausal women also raises the level of vitamin D in the bloodstream and increases intestinal calcium absorption. Therefore, there is some evidence that a fall in active vitamin D levels, possibly because of a fall in vitamin D production due to aging or estrogen deficiency, may account for some of the decrease in intestinal calcium absorption with age. Also, the aging intestine may become somewhat resistant to the action of vitamin D, and this may result in less calcium absorption.

Most studies of vitamin D levels in postmenopausal women have found them to be normal. But elderly women who do not get much exposure to sunlight have been found to be slightly deficient in vitamin D. Their deficiency may be due to reduced production of vitamin D. Usually we are not vitamin D deficient because we obtain enough vitamin D from sunlight, which is then converted to an active form in the liver and the kidney. However, vitamin D deficiency does occur in persons who usually stay indoors or are severely malnourished.

Vitamin D Supplements in Treating Osteoporosis

Still, studies have focused on vitamin D supplements as a treatment for osteoporosis. In one study, over 3200 French women about 84 years of age who were in nursing homes were randomized to take either 800 IU per day of vitamin D (equivalent to the amount in two multiple vitamins a day) and a 500-milligram calcium supplement or no treatment. At the end of the 18-month study, the women treated with the vitamin D and calcium had an increase in bone density of the hip and a 40 percent reduction in hip fractures compared to the group that was not treated. All of the study subjects had evidence of low bone formation and had low blood levels of vitamin D. The reduction in hip fractures was dramatic, showing that calcium absorption and vitamin D actions are severely impaired in the very elderly. Since calcium is critical to bone mass, any problem with calcium absorption would compromise bone; the simple addition of vitamin D increased calcium absorption, which may have increased the bone mass in these women. Also, vitamin D may have increased the activity of the osteoblasts, the cells that form bone. So, a small dose of vitamin D and calcium together dramatically reduced the risk of fractures in these women.

Another interesting discovery about vitamin D and bone mass in the elderly is that in the winter months in Boston, Massachusetts, vertebral bone mass fell; vitamin D levels also fell in postmenopausal women who were taking about 100 IU a day of this vitamin. When these women were given 400 IU per day of a vitamin D supplement, the amount found in a standard multiple vitamin, this wintertime bone loss was prevented. Therefore, these two studies demonstrate how mild vitamin D deficiency or calcium deficiency can be easily corrected, resulting in a dramatic reduction in fractures and prevention of bone loss.

On the other hand, when men and women who were already taking the RDAs of vitamin D and calcium were given supplements, no preservation of bone mass was seen. Preservation of bone mass and prevention of fractures in the elderly seem to occur only when the person does not take in enough calcium and vitamin D.

Other studies have been done using 1,25 dihydroxyvitamin D to treat postmenopausal women with osteoporosis. In one study done in New Zealand, postmenopausal women who had at least one osteoporotic fracture were randomly given either 1,25 dihydroxyvitamin D or calcium. The women who were given the vitamin had fewer new vertebral and nonvertebral fractures than those who were given calcium. The investigators believed that vitamin D worked and was safe for the treatment of postmenopausal osteoporosis.

Still other studies have been done to determine if 1,25 dihydroxyvitamin D can be used to treat osteoporosis in the United States. These studies differed from others because the dose of vitamin D and the amount of daily dietary calcium were adjusted to prevent serum and urinary calcium levels from getting too high, and the dose of vitamin D was smaller. All the subjects were postmenopausal and had at least one vertebral fracture when they entered the study. No study showed a change in the fracture rate or bone turnover, as measured by bone biopsies, or any increase in vertebral or forearm bone mass. Other studies found high serum and urine calcium levels while the subjects were taking vitamin D.

In general, the few studies that have been done found that 1,25 dihydroxyvitamin D appears to decrease the rate of new fractures and stabilizes, if not slightly increases, bone mass. It can be used to treat osteoporosis if adequate doses are used. Unfortunately, the doses required to treat osteoporosis dramatically increase serum and urine calcium levels, so that the margin of safety with this medication is narrow.

An exciting advance in the use of vitamin D to prevent or treat osteoporosis is the development of vitamin D analogues. These medications are very similar in chemical structure and activity to natural vitamin D. One benefit of vitamin D analogues is that they seem to be able to increase calcium absorption from the intestine, and some of them work without raising the blood or urine calcium to dangerous levels. Further research may lead to the development of these medications for the treatment of osteoporosis.

VITAMIN D AND SKELETAL DEVELOPMENT

Vitamin D supplementation is also important in the development of the skeleton. Growing children, whose bone mass is increasing, need vitamin D to increase calcium absorption, to allow normal mineralization of bone, and to help the osteoblast cells that form bone to mature. When a child is ill and housebound for a long time, or takes a medication that prevents normal bone growth like steroids or anticancer drugs, the addition of supplemental vitamin D to their diet is essential. Although studies are now going on to determine more precisely how vitamin D supplements should be used to promote bone mass development in children, we can safely say that every child should obtain at least 400 IU per day in the form of a multiple vitamin; in fact, 800 IU per day or two multiple vitamins is preferred.

Vitamin D, like vitamins A, E, and K, is fat soluble. This means that its absorption by the body depends somewhat on how well the person absorbs fat. Diseases or conditions that impair fat absorption, like celiac sprue (poor absorption of nutrients from the stomach and intestines), prior gastric surgery, or inflammatory bowel disease, may reduce the absorption of fat-soluble vitamins. These people may become deficient in vitamin D, and because this vitamin is needed for calcium absorption, they may also become deficient in calcium later on. They must be sure to go outdoors to obtain the vitamin D that they need from sunlight; they must also take multiple vitamins. Even in someone who has a problem absorbing fat, if vitamin D is taken in the form of a multiple vitamin, more of it will be absorbed.

THE GENETICS OF OSTEOPOROSIS

An exciting breakthrough in recent years is our improved understanding of the genetics of osteoporosis. This work has pinpointed a group of women with a certain vitamin D receptor, a protein on the cell surface that binds with vitamin D that does not work correctly. Some women with this receptor, called BB, have trouble absorbing calcium from the gastrointestinal tract, and thus they have low bone mass for their age and sex. Since we inherit a gene for the vitamin D receptor from each parent, our genetic profile can be normal, abnormal, or somewhere in between. So, genetic heritage seems to point to an identifiable cause of inherited osteoporosis or low bone mass. In a few years, we will find that it is many genes together that contribute to osteoporosis. Although one of them may be the vitamin D receptor gene, this gene seems to increase the risk of developing osteoporosis by only about twofold. Calcium absorption when we are growing is also important to achieve peak bone mass. Calcium absorption becomes important again around the age of 80 years, when our ability to absorb it decreases and a negative calcium balance develops. Therefore, defects in the vitamin D receptor gene may prevent certain persons from achieving peak bone mass, and these persons may lose more bone mass in old age. At this time, this new information can only be interpreted as interesting, and the vitamin D receptor gene is probably only one of the many genetic components of osteoporosis. Also, taking a normal amount of vitamin D or a little extra calcium could probably override any of the calcium deficiency in these individuals and could probably make up for any defects in the action of vitamin D. Much more work is needed to figure out how this genetic trait fits into osteoporosis because, in some populations, the BB gene increases the risk of developing osteoporosis about twofold, but in other populations it does not increase this risk at all. There is probably a lot more to the story.

SUMMARY

- Vitamin D is essential for bone health. It promotes calcium intake and maturation of bone cells.
- Vitamin D supplementation comes from sunlight, multiple vitamins, vegetables, and special vitamin D formulations.
- Other than low-dose supplementation, there is no direct role for vitamin D in the prevention and treatment of osteoporosis.

9

Exercise, Bone Health, and Osteoporosis

Probably no area of medical research has received as much interest in recent years as exercise. Indeed, it has been well documented that 30 minutes of exercise three or four times a week will prevent heart disease. However, exercise also has many positive effects on our bones.

Our bones respond to stresses and strains. When we exercise, our muscles stress the bones, and the bones remodel and become stronger. The cortical bone, or the outer envelope of bone, is probably most responsive to exercise-induced changes because it lies next to the muscles. We also know that the best exercises to put stress on the skeleton and induce bone formation are weight-bearing exercises. What we do not yet know is what the best exercise prescription is, what types of exercise are best, and how often and how intense they need to be to obtain peak bone mass.

EXERCISE AND BONE MASS

Exercise and bone mass studies generally show that men and women who perform weight-bearing exercise three to five times a week generally have slightly more bone mass than those who do not exercise. Typical weight-bearing exercises include jogging, running, brisk walking, weight lifting, and team and individual sports like basketball, baseball, or tennis. But when we try to find out if exercise will build bone or prevent bone loss in menopausal or elderly women, we must conduct a prospective study; that is, one that follows the study subjects over time. When a prospective study was done in premenopausal women in their 30s and 40s, weight-lifting exercises resulted in an increase in lumbar spine bone mineral density of less than 1 percent a year. Another study of weight training in women found no increase in lumbar bone density after a year.

On the other hand, when college women who were not physically active were entered into a study of calcium and exercise, there was a 3 to 5 percent increase in lumbar bone mineral density after 1 year in the women who had been in the exercise group of the study. The results of this study are different from those of other prospective studies of exercise and bone mass. The women who entered this study had to be rather inactive; that is, they could not have participated in regular exercise programs beforehand. Then, once they started to exercise, new stress or increased stress was placed on their bones, and the bones remodeled, strengthened, and increased in mass. In other studies, women were probably already fairly active, so the new exercise regimen, even if it included weight-lifting exercises, still did not create enough new strain for the bones to remodel and increase in mass. The level of stress on the skeleton from exercise must be greater than usual or no real changes will occur.

EXERCISE IN THE OLDER ADULT

A study of elderly women living in a nursing home found that isometric exercises three to five times a week increased lumbar bone mass over 3 percent in 8 months; the increases were highest in those women who had been least active before the exercise program began.

EXERCISE IN WOMEN OF CHILDBEARING AGE

About the age of 30, men and women achieve peak bone mass. From ages 30 to 50, bone mass in women remains stable.

Exercises that build muscle strength, like weight lifting or weight-bearing exercises such as jogging, brisk walking, aerobic dance, tap dancing, jazz dancing, or tennis strengthen the muscles of the back, arms, and legs and maintain or slightly increase bone mass. Exercises that strengthen the muscles put stress on the bones, which then triggers the bones to remodel. Bone is then added to adapt to the higher stresses that the exercise creates. Usually these changes occur in the cortical bone next to the muscles.

The types of exercise that can increase bone mass in a woman of childbearing age include jogging, running, brisk walking, weight lifting, stair-step walking, treadmill walking and jogging, tennis, racquetball, basketball, and soccer. The types of exercise that do not increase bone mass include swimming, walking, gardening, outdoor bicycling, and stationary exercise bicycling.

The bone mass in the spine and hips usually increases slightly with weight-bearing exercises. The less active a woman is when she begins an exercise program, the more likely it is that she will gain bone mass. If a woman who does not exercise starts an exercise program of brisk walking and carrying hand weights three or four times a week for 30 minutes, she may experience a 3 to 5 percent increase in lumbar spine bone mass after a year. A woman who is already active usually does not gain much bone mass from additional exercise because her bones have already adapted to the increased stresses of exercise.

Once a woman starts an exercise program, as long as the exercise regimen is continued at the same intensity, the bone gain will remain. However, if the exercise is stopped or the amount of time spent exercising is reduced, bone mass will also decrease.

We do not know how much exercise is needed to increase bone mass in this age group. However, 30 minutes of exercise, three to four times a week is probably sufficient. The exercise should be intense enough to build up a sweat. This type of exercise should be adequate to maintain or slightly increase bone mass in women during the childbearing years.

Excessive Exercise in Women of Childbearing Age and Middle Age

Moderate exercise is fine for bone, but excessive exercising leads to extreme weight loss, and menstrual cycles become lighter or stop; this signals that the estrogen level is low, and bone loss can occur. Often this bone loss results in a stress fracture of the foot or lower leg. The stress fractures due to low bone mass resemble those of older osteoporotic women. These fractures usually heal without complications. However, this is a sign that a woman has low bone mass. She should reduce her exercise regimen until her menstrual periods return, and she should take calcium supplements to try to restore the bone mass lost while her menstrual periods stopped. Although, this is not often mentioned, overexercise, loss of menstrual periods, and bone loss is also a problem in middle-aged women and signals osteoporosis before menopause. Therefore, exercise in middle-aged women should be monitored, keeping it below the level that creates abnormal menstrual periods or *amenorrhea* (loss of the menstrual cycle).

Exercise After Prolonged Inactivity to Rebuild Bone Mass

Women who have been confined to bed for any length of time because of surgery or a long illness will experience some bone loss. Exercise can strengthen muscles and restore the lost bone. Initially, the exercise program should emphasize muscle strengthening and endurance. After muscle strength is recovered, weight-bearing exercises and exercises of higher intensity can be done.

It may take a year or more to increase bone mass. However, the other health-related benefits of exercise, like weight reduction, increased muscle strength, increased sense of well-being, reduced blood pressure, and reduced cholesterol level, can be felt almost immediately.

Does Exercise During the Childbearing Years Prevent Osteoporosis?

Moderate weight-bearing and resistance exercises between the ages of 30 and 50 years will increase a woman's bone mass. This will provide additional bone mass when she enters menopause so that she will have more bone to lose before she develops osteoporosis and fractures in her later years.

Exercise and Estrogen as a Treatment Strategy

A very exciting study was done in women in early menopause to determine if estrogen and exercise would help maintain bone mass. Menopausal women were assigned to either an estrogen-only group, exercise alone three times a week with resistance training, or estrogen replacement plus a three-times-a week resistance-training program. After 1 year, lumbar spine bone mineral density was unchanged in the estrogen-only group, increased about 8 percent in the estrogen and exercise group, and increased about 4 percent in the exercise-alone group. This study was the first to show that the bone mineral density of the lumbar spine increases with resistance training. So, exercise may help to slow bone loss in early menopause but for real gain in bone mass to occur, estrogen therapy is necessary as well.

Another study found that a 1-year walking program had no effect on bone mineral density of the lumbar spine. In still another study, elderly women were placed in groups with either aerobic exercise alone or both aerobic exercise and strength training, or in a control group. After 1 year, both of the exercising groups obtained small increases in bone mass (4 to 8 percent); the control group did not.

The effect of short-term exercise and detraining (stopping an exercise program) on lumbar spine bone mineral density was estimated from a study done on 35 postmenopausal women. These women were placed randomly in either an exercise group or a control group. The exercise group had three exercise sessions per week, including 50 to 60 minutes of walking, jogging, stair climbing, and light resistance training. After 9 months, bone mineral density of the lumbar spine increased modestly (about 6 percent) in the exercise group and decreased slightly in the control group. However, 13 months after the exercise group stopped exercising, their bone mineral content returned to only 1 percent above the baseline (beginning or first) value. This tells us that exercise must be continued indefinitely for bone mineral improvement to persist in elderly women.

EXERCISE IN WOMEN WITH OSTEOPOROSIS

Very few studies have looked at the effect of exercise on women with established osteoporosis. One study focused on women aged 50 to 73 who had sustained a Colles' fracture (affecting the forearm or wrist). These women took part in a general aerobic exercise program for 8 months. Lumbar spine bone mass increased modestly (about 3 percent) in the exercise group and decreased by the same amount in the nonexercise group. Another study involved an exercise program designed to improve the functional abilities of patients with osteoporosis and to provide social interaction. The subjects' compliance with this program was high, and their aerobic capacity and bone mass increased dramatically. Also, no fractures occurred. This was important because some physicians are reluctant to prescribe exercise for women with osteoporotic fractures out of fear of additional injuries or another fracture. In fact, *avoiding* activity is harmful. It accelerates the decline of the musculoskeletal system and increases the risk of developing another fracture.

Studies of exercise in women with fractures of the spine generally found that resistance exercises designed to strengthen the back extensors reduced the development of new vertebral fractures. However, exercises designed to strengthen back flexors increased vertebral deformities and fractures. Therefore, in women with osteoporosis of the spine, it appears that activities that place too much stress on the front of the spine, as in flexing a muscle, are particularly risky, and patients must be taught to avoid it. Rehabilitation after a fracture is discussed in Chapter 12.

While exercise may produce only small gains in bone mass, if any, it may reduce other risk factors for fractures. In particular, it may improve muscle strength, flexibility, balance, and posture, thereby reducing the risk of falling and decreasing the severity of the fall. Because over 90 percent of hip fractures are the result of a fall, anything that reduces the rate of falling and the severity of the fall may greatly reduce hip fractures.

Although we know very little about the best exercises for maximizing bone mass after 70, a few recommendations are possible. Most important, the exercise program should not be harmful. It should increase the person's ability to perform day-to-day activities and minimize the risk of later fractures. Thus, for persons who have not exercised before, the program must be of low intensity and must emphasize safety. A gradual progression of exercise intensity may reduce injuries and will encourage the person to continue exercising. Also, for the increase in bone mass to be sustained, the exercise must be continued indefinitely and may even have to be intensified continuously. The exercise program should also avoid loading the weak part of the body. Women with spine fractures, for example, must avoid exercises that require backward bending. For these women, the dangers of lifting when flexing must also be emphasized. Exercise programs should concentrate on gradually increasing the strength of the back extensor muscles—the muscles that can prevent future fractures.

Remember, exercise is not a daily activity in most adults. Any exercise that an elderly person does continuously must be simple and enjoyable enough to accommodate the individual with average motivation, limited access to special exercise equipment, and a busy schedule.

IMPORTANCE OF THE TYPE OF EXERCISE PERFORMED

We have found that the *kind* of exercise used is important because the stress or load on the skeleton from the exercise makes a difference in how the bone will respond. A low-impact or loading exercise, like brisk walking, does not add much stress to the skeleton and thus does not increase bone mass much at all. The same is true of swimming. Although swimming is a very good exercise for cardiovascular conditioning, it does not increase bone mass (see Table 9.1).

While researchers are still working to determine which types of exercise are best for preventing bone loss, we do know the time of life at which exercise is critical for bone mass. Exercise can make a big difference in young adults aged 13–30 years in preventing osteoporosis. When the skeleton is still maturing and adding bone during this period, regular weight-bearing exercise and good calcium intake

Table 9.1. *Exercise and Bone Mass*

*Examples of exercises that can maintain bone mass and muscle strength
in women in their childbearing years and in menopause*

Aerobic or energy-burning exercises	Swimming
Vigorous walking, hiking	Racket sports
Jogging or brisk walking	Gardening that works up a sweat
Aerobic dance, jazzercise	Cross-country skiing
Bicycling—both outdoors and stationary	Weight lifting or working out in a gym
Jumping rope	

Less energy-burning stretching exercises

Dance	Stretching
Yoga	

can increase peak bone mass. The higher the peak bone mass, the more bone mass must be lost before the person risks developing an osteoporotic fracture.

And yet, while regular, moderate exercise can do a lot to prevent osteoporosis by increasing peak bone mass in young adults, exercise to prevent bone loss in women after menopause is not especially beneficial. However, if a woman is not very active or lived in a nursing facility, she can benefit from exercise and even develop some new bone. But these gains from exercise will not be maintained unless the exercise is continued.

In 1984 we began a study at the Stanford Arthritis Center focusing on female runners about 60 years of age who ran for 9 years, about 3–4 miles a day, for about 200 minutes a week. The bone mineral density of the lumbar spine in these women, when first measured, was 20 percent higher than that of a control group of nonrunners. When we measured the bone mineral density again 2 years later, the runners had decreased their running time per week by 25 percent to about 150 minutes, and their bone mineral density had decreased by about 16 percent. When we looked again at these women 5 years into the study, the runners had again decreased their running time and a similar decrease in bone mass had occurred. From these findings, we can draw several conclusions. When we reach adulthood, after the time of peak bone mass development at age 30, we cannot put bone in the bank and draw interest on it. The body is too smart for that. Bone mass will respond to the stresses upon it, but if the stresses decrease, bone will remodel and bone mass will decrease. If the stresses increase, bone will remodel and bone mass will increase to some extent.

So, while exercise is important to our health as adults, the overall benefits for bone mass are relatively minor. Exercise does not prevent estrogen-deficient bone loss.

SPECIAL PROBLEMS OF THE FEMALE ATHLETE

Women of all ages are becoming increasingly involved in athletic activities at both the recreational and competitive levels. Although there are numerous benefits to physical activity, specific problems may occur in the various stages of a female athlete's life, especially with reproduction, which then affects her bones. Delayed sexual maturation in the adolescent athlete and abnormal or absent menstrual cycles in the adult woman are some of the concerns. Other major problems include eating disorders, skeletal abnormalities that result from reduced bone density, stress fractures, and failure to achieve peak bone mass associated with amenorrhea, or loss of the menstrual cycle. Since many of these issues concern the adolescent athlete and since they affect her bone mass for life, we will consider her first.

The Adolescent Athlete

Strenuous physical activity has a profound effect on the sexual maturation of the adolescent athlete. It has long been known that the age of *menarche* (the start of menstruation) is later in athletes compared to nonathletes. And this delay occurs more often in activities in which the athletes are thin, such as ballet dancing, gymnastics, running, and figure skating. In fact, some dancers and runners do not have their first menstrual period until their 20s.

Menarche is only one event in puberty. It is not yet clear whether all stages of puberty are delayed because few studies have addressed this question. Ballet dancers have delayed menarche, delayed breast development, and delayed bone age; the development of pubic hair is not affected. In gymnasts, both breast and pubic hair development are delayed by about a year or two compared to swimmers and non-athletic schoolgirls. The mechanism of delayed puberty in these athletes is not completely understood, but normal puberty occurs when gonadotropin-releasing hormone (GNRH) enters the bloodstream and stimulates luteinizing hormone (LH) secretion from the pituitary. In the late-maturing athlete, lack of GNRH suppresses LH secretion.

The results of delayed puberty on these young athletes are not completely known. Low bone mineral density is one of the major consequences, and it has been reported in athletes with exercise-associated amenorrhea. Bone mass accretion, which normally occurs during adolescence, is reduced in these later-maturing girls because of the absence of estrogen. If there is no gain in bone mass during adolescence, the athlete's peak bone mass may not be obtained, and the relative *osteopenia* (low bone mass) may result in a higher risk of injury. Indeed, more than half of ballet dancers who had delayed menarche developed a stress fracture during their training. *Scoliosis*, or curvature of the spine, is also more frequent in ballet dancers with delayed menarche. The end result of delayed menarche is that these women enter menopause with a substantially lower bone mass than normal women.

If an adolescent athlete has delayed menarche, she should have a thorough workup by a physician who is experienced in adolescent growth and development. Both pediatric endocrinologists and some obstetrician-gynecologists who specialize in adolescent development are the appropriate physicians to consult. Important information for the physician to obtain includes the athlete's training intensity, eating habits, history of growth and development, and the blood levels of hormones, including LH, follicle-stimulating hormone (FSH), estradiol, and thyroid hormones.

Usually, treatment will depend on the athlete's age and stage of puberty, and whether she has complications such as low bone density or stress fractures. These young athletes should be encouraged to decrease the intensity of their training or exercise and to improve their nutritional intake, since rest and weight gain often allow them to catch up and experience puberty. If a young woman has not reached menarche by the age of 16, estrogen therapy may be started under a physician's supervision. This therapy increases bone mass, which does not happen normally in the adolescent girl with a low estrogen level. Generally, she must remain on estrogen indefinitely.

The long-term effects of delayed puberty on growth and development are not known. It is believed that delayed menarche prevents young women from achieving peak bone mass and predisposes the adolescent athlete to skeletal fragility that could result in osteoporosis.

Effect on the Reproductive System in Adult Athletes

Several menstrual irregularities have been described in adult women athletes. These problem occur often in sports in which the athletes are thin and the training is intense—usually less than 5 percent in the nonathletic population. The prevalence of menstrual irregularities in ballet dancers is consistently high; in cyclists and swimmers, the incidence is the same as that of the normal population. One result of menstrual dysfunction in adult athletes is osteoporosis; others include infertility, abnormal cholesterol or lipid metabolism, and coronary artery disease. We will now discuss osteoporosis.

Osteoporosis and other skeletal problems related to low bone mass, or osteopenia, have become a focus of concern in athletes whose menstrual cycles have ceased. Many factors influence the amount of bone in female athletes, including the type and duration of the menstrual irregularities (having fewer menstrual periods, shortened and/ or lighter bleeding in menstrual cycles), the hormones present in the blood, the amount of weight-bearing exercise that the athlete is doing, the weight changes during training, the amount of body fat, and the nutritional intake, especially of calcium.

Women in general tend to lose about 1 percent of their bone mass a year from early in their 30s on, whereas athletes who no longer have menstrual periods appear to lose about 5 percent of their bone mass per year. The rate of bone loss in amenorrheic women is similar to that in women who are in early menopause. The loss is mainly in the trabecular (interior) bone, so the changes in bone mass are most obvious in the lumbar spine, the pelvis, and the upper femurs around the hip. Trabecular bone has a high turnover rate and is most sensitive to changes in estrogen level. Changes in trabecular bone mass occur within months of amenorrhea. By contrast, changes in cortical bone with amenorrhea can take years. One study of female amenorrheic athletes found that the bone mineral density of the lumbar spine was lower than that of a 50-year-old woman. The areas of the body with more cortical bone are less affected initially by the amenorrhea-associated bone loss because the turnover rate of cortical bone is much slower.

Estrogen deficiency, which plays a critical role in the loss of bone mass after menopause, is the main cause of osteopenia in both young women and premenopausal amenorrheic athletes. Absence of estrogen during adolescence or at any time during the premenopausal years will decrease bone density. Therefore, the low level of estrogen that results in amenorrhea in premenopausal women athletes reduces bone mass—which becomes a lifelong problem.

Amenorrhea in premenopausal women may lead to irreversible bone loss. A study of amenorrheic athletes in their 20s who resumed their menstrual cycles found that these women had an increase in bone mineral density of their lumbar spine and about about half as much again the following year. But then no increase was observed for the next 2 years. So it seems that women athletes who experience amenorrhea will have some spinal bone loss. If their menstrual periods resume, they will regain some of the lost bone mass, but their lumbar bone density will probably be permanently lower than that of women who have always had a normal cycle.

The amenorrheic athlete has a low estrogen level. This results in loss of bone mass and increases her risk of developing stress fractures. Regular exercise is important in preventing heart disease because it decreases LDL (bad) cholesterol and increases HDL (good) cholesterol. Unfortunately, the beneficial effects of regular strenuous exercise on heart disease may be reversed by exercise-induced amenorrhea. The estrogen that normally reduces the LDL level is decreased in these women. As a result, cholesterol levels can increase in young women with amenorrhea. Whether this will increase their risk of coronary artery disease is unknown, but it is definitely a potential problem and a good reason for these women to avoid prolonged amenorrhea.

While exercise helps to reduce the rate of normal bone loss that occurs in postmenopausal women, it does not protect the amenorrheic young athlete. On the contrary: The increased bone mineral density in weight-bearing bone that is usually seen with exercise is not found in amenorrheic dancers and runners. In fact, amenorrheic athletes lost over 3 percent of their spinal bone mineral density over the 15 months they were followed in a study, despite a regular exercise program, while athletes with a normal menstrual cycle lost no bone mass. Nevertheless, exercise is somewhat important in the amenorrheic athlete because sedentary amenorrheic athletes lose more bone mass than actively exercising amenorrheic athletes.

Female athletes also frequently have eating disorders. It has long been known that food deprivation can lead to menstrual abnormalities and low bone mass as an adult.

In a study of weight control behavior in female athletes, it was found that about one-fourth of the 182 varsity-level athletes used diet pills routinely, about 15 percent used laxatives, and a small percentage used self-induced vomiting. The percentage of women who restrained their eating, did binge-purge eating, and used self-induced vomiting varied among different sports. Of the women who do not participate in athletics, around 5 percent have an eating disorder. Athletes who participate in sports where leanness is emphasized very often have eating disorders. Ballet dancers have the most, about 30 percent; gymnasts, around 70 percent; and track runners, about 30 percent. Among athletes who participate in sports where leanness is not emphasized, including tennis, volleyball, and swimming, the proportion of women with eating disorders is about 20 percent. Although these results reflect only a few studies, they show that eating disorders are common in these young female athletes, and that when they do not eat right and are thin, they can develop menstrual irregularities, have fewer menstrual periods, or develop amenorrhea—all of which lead to bone loss.

We also know that poor nutrition in their early 20s will prevent young athletes from achieving high peak bone mass even if they do not develop menstrual abnormalities. Therefore, poor nutrition and low calcium intake are just two of the factors that influence bone mass in female athletes.

Stress Fractures: Osteoporosis in Young and Middle-Aged Athletes

As we have seen, female athletes with low bone density can develop stress fractures. These fractures may result from overuse of bones that are weak due to osteopenia. Stress fractures occur among dancers and runners who are amenorrheic or who have a history of menstrual abnormalities. The ones at highest risk of stress fractures are those who have had menstrual irregularities for a long time. Runners with menstrual abnormalities tend to have multiple stress fractures. The cause of the fractures is not completely clear, but repetitive stress and trauma on the bone, say from running, and the stress superimposed by fragile bones can increase the risk. We can think of a stress fracture in an athlete as an "overuse" injury; the stresses put on bone that is already thin are too great, and the bone collapses. The bone mass cannot withstand the forces that are continually put on it.

But we learned earlier that bone can remodel and increase its mass when the stresses placed on it are greater than normal; conversely, bone mass will decrease when the stresses placed on it are decreased. With stress fracture, the bone is unable to remodel fast enough to increase its mass to support the increased load. Stress fractures tend to occur not only in female athletes with menstrual abnormalities, but also in athletes who have increased too quickly either the time or the intensity of their activity. The bones most commonly fractured include the fibula (small bone of the lower leg), the metatarsals (small bones in the foot), the tibia (large bone of the lower leg), and the femur (large bone of the thigh).

A recent study asked 300 female collegiate track runners at over 20 colleges in the United States to fill out a questionnaire about their training habits, menstrual histories, medications, and injury history. The results showed that many of them had a delay in menarche if they had started intense training before their menstrual periods began. Also, many of them had eating disorders, consuming fewer than 1000 calories a day of all foods, even though they were training intensively. During the year preceding the study, many of them had experienced stress fractures; the areas most commonly fractured included the bones of the lower leg, foot, and midfoot, the heel bone, and even the thigh and pelvic bones—about 180 stress fractures in all. The risk of a stress fracture was increased in the young women who were having fewer than three menstrual periods a year, had started regular athletic training more than a year before they had their first menstrual period, and had eating disorders. What is interesting is that the amenorrheic runners who were taking birth control pills had a decreased risk of developing a stress fracture. Since birth control pills contain both estrogen and progesterone, these women were still receiving enough of these hormones from the pills to protect them against fractures. Unfortunately, there is no prospective study of these women from the time they first start taking birth control pills to measure their bone mass, how much they eat, and their level of cholesterol. This information would be very important for the women, their parents, and their athletic coaches.

Today young women start intensive athletic training very young, well before their first menstrual period. The intensity of the training delays menarche at the appropriate time, which, in turn, delays the development of bone mass usually seen at this stage of life. This delay may prevent these women from achieving the peak bone mass they otherwise would have developed. The low bone mass in these young women will greatly increase their chances of developing osteoporosis and fractures throughout their athletic careers.

These women athletes also have eating disorders and cut down on calories, hurting their chances of achieving and maintaining healthy bones. And even when these women do go through menarche, if they continue to train at a very competitive level, they may not have a regular monthly menstrual cycle, may have few menstrual periods a year (*oligomenorrhea*), or may develop secondary amenorrhea and stop menstruating completely. All of these conditions are associated with low estrogen levels and bone loss.

The development of amenorrhea in a young woman is just like menopause in a 50-year-old woman. The estrogen level drops by at least 50 percent, and both young and old women lose bone. This is a serious problem because the young woman, who has never achieved her peak bone mass, is already losing bone.

The young athlete who takes birth control pills appears to be able to prevent some of this bone loss, but she still may not achieve peak bone mass and may never regain the bone mass she has lost. The woman going through menopause can choose to take estrogen to prevent bone loss, and this will prevent her from developing osteoporosis.

What Recommendations Are Sensible Given Our Current Knowledge?

A young woman should probably not begin intense physical training until she has had her first menstrual period, and she probably should monitor the amount and intensity of the exercise until her menstrual periods are normal. These two practices alone will allow the increase in bone mass that occurs with puberty and will allow her body to get used to normal circulating estrogen levels. The intensively training young athlete should be counseled about the long-term risks of this training. She should be encouraged to use birth control pills to increase her estrogen level, and she should probably be advised to train less intensively. If she is not eating well, she should be counseled about a balanced diet and the risks of not eating well.

An important point to remember is that when an amenorrheic woman stops training due to an injury or another problem, she usually gains some weight and regains her menstrual periods. With the return of menstrual periods she can regain bone mass, but none of the women studied to date have gained back all the bone mass they have lost. Nor do they develop normal bone mass for their age. In fact, some of this damage may never be repaired, and the need for education and prevention is painfully apparent. Today, luckily, amenorrhea, eating disorders, and stress fractures appear to be limited to the sports that require trim bodies, primarily running, track, gymnastics, and dance. Where the emphasis on leanness is less important, in tennis, volleyball, and swimming, eating disorders, amenorrhea, delayed menarche, and stress fractures seem to be less problematic. But we must be cautious in making these distinctions between different sports because not enough research has been done to determine if the distinction is real. Also, as young women become more involved in sports, the intensity of training in every sport may have the same consequences.

SUMMARY

- Men and women who perform weight-bearing exercise three to five times a week generally have more bone mass than nonexercisers.
- Elderly persons who perform aerobic or isometric exercises may have a modest (few percent) increase in the bone mass of the lumbar spine. This exercise must be performed regularly for bone mass to be maintained.
- In persons with osteoporosis, exercise increases lumbar bone mass slightly. It also increases muscle strength, flexibility, balance, and posture, reducing the risk of falling and fractures.
- Exercise for women of childbearing age that increases muscle strength triggers bone remodeling, increasing bone mass.
- A combination of exercise and estrogen therapy is necessary to build bone in early menopause.
- Excessive exercise in women of childbearing age and middle age leads to extreme weight loss, as well as lightening of the menstrual cycle or amenorrhea. This indicates a low estrogen level, and bone loss, possibly with fractures, can occur.
- Prolonged bed rest leads to loss of bone. Exercise should be done first to strengthen the muscles and increase endurance. Then weight-bearing and higher-intensity exercises should be done.
- In the adolescent athlete, menarche is often delayed. Bone mass is lost and peak bone mass may not be obtained, increasing the risk of injury. Training and exercise should be decreased and food intake increased so that puberty can occur.
- Adult female athletes may have menstrual irregularities or amenorrhea, which may lead to low bone mass, osteoporosis, and infertility, among other problems. They may also have eating disorders. These conditions lead to low peak bone mass and stress fractures.
- Young women should probably delay intense physical training until after menarche. Exercise should be monitored until men-

strual periods are normal. Good nutrition is important. Birth control pills increase the estrogen level and prevent bone loss.

MARGIE: LOW BONE MINERAL DENSITY AND A FAMILY HISTORY OF OSTEOPOROSIS

Margie is a 36-year-old white woman who is 5 feet 3 inches tall and weighs 100 pounds. She has one child and a strong family history of osteoporosis; both her mother and her father's sister developed osteoporotic compression fractures of the spine in their early 70s. Margie is a competitive runner and runs over 60 miles a week in training. Last year she developed a stress fracture of her first metatarsal bone (a small bone in her midfoot), which her doctor said resulted from running too much. Over the past 2 years she has not had a menstrual period (secondary amenorrhea). Her calcium intake is about 900 milligrams a day, obtained from her diet and a calcium supplement.

Margie's physician recently decided to measure her bone mass. The BMD of her spine is 0.82 g/cm^2. Her T score is -2.5, which means that she already has osteoporosis.

Margie reached her peak bone mass at about the age of 30. Now, 6 years later, her bone is already reduced. Her condition may be genetic or may stem from the overtraining that has led to the secondary amenorrhea, lowered her estrogen level, and caused further loss of bone mass. A combination of both factors is the most likely explanation.

This is a difficult case because much of the damage has already been done. Nothing can be done about Margie's genetic predisposition to osteoporosis or about her reaching bone maturity with low bone mass. Margie must focus now on preventing the loss of any more bone.

Secondary amenorrhea is not uncommon in athletes who train hard. It is especially common in women who participate in sports that emphasize thinness, like running and gymnastics. But amenorrhea results in a low estrogen level, which causes amenorrheic women, like menopausal women, to lose bone mass. At this time, Margie should have her amenorrhea evaluated.

Margie must decrease the intensity of her training and gain some weight; with these steps, her menstrual cycle should return. Until that time, Margie should consider taking birth control pills. These contain a combination of estrogen and progesterone, and the estrogen should be enough to prevent further loss of bone while she is amenorrheic. Margie must work with her physician, either a general physician or an obstetrician-gynecologist, to find the right birth control pill for her.

If Margie will not take a birth control pill and will not reduce the intensity of her training, she must consider taking another medication that will prevent her from losing any more bone mass; two choices are alendronate (a bisphosphonate) and intranasal calcitonin. Neither of these medications is approved for the prevention of bone loss in premenopausal women, but in this case they should be considered.

Margie must also consider her future because her reduced bone mass puts her at high risk of developing osteoporotic fractures. While Margie is amenorrheic, it is very important for her to increase her daily calcium intake. Usually the estrogen in the body helps to absorb calcium from the gastrointestinal tract. Since Margie's estrogen level is as low as a postmenopausal woman's, she needs the same amount of calcium as a postmenopausal woman. So, through a combination of diet and supplements, Margie must increase her calcium intake to 1500 milligrams a day. In addition, a multiple vitamin that contains about 400 IU of vitamin D is needed to help her absorb the calcium. Margie's current intake of calcium is 900 milligrams a day, so she needs to add 600 milligrams. She can easily do this by taking a supplement of calcium carbonate or calcium gluconate.

Today we do not know much about women like Margie, who, 15 years before menopause, is already osteoporotic. What we do know is that her low bone density puts her at very high risk of developing more fractures as she ages. Physicians try to encourage these women to try to regain their menstrual periods and to take birth control pills until they go through menopause. When Margie regains her menstrual periods, she will regain some of the bone mass lost during amenorrhea, but she will not regain it all. Women like Margie will probably be candidates for bone-building medications when they become available for general use, but until that time, all of Margie's efforts should be directed at preventing further bone loss.

10

Bone-Building Agents: Are There Any "Magic Bullets"?

When we describe osteoporosis, we describe a disease of low bone mass and low bone strength. This condition occurs most frequently in elderly women after many years of menopause and low estrogen levels. The hallmark of osteoporosis is fractures from very low trauma at the hip and the vertebrae of the spine. Hip fractures create the most immediate financial stress and physical suffering. Most persons who suffer a hip fracture need surgery; an estimated one-sixth of these patients die within 3 months, and nearly half of all of the others suffer some functional decline. Vertebral fractures, on the other hand, have few symptoms and contribute to an often silent decline in an individual's quality of life.

Current treatments for osteoporosis focus on reducing bone loss by slowing the bone remodeling cycle. These treatments work for a few years to increase bone mass by a small amount. Treatment of an osteoporotic woman with alendronate results in a 2–6 percent increase in bone mass over the first 3 years; similar findings have been reported with estrogen replacement therapy. But an increase in bone mass of 2–6 percent over a 3-year period will probably do little for a woman who has had osteoporotic fractures and whose bone mass is 35 percent below her peak bone mass. This woman needs much more bone mass and improved bone structure to avoid future fractures. Currently, the agents used to treat or prevent osteoporosis—estrogen, bisphosphonates, calcitonin, calcium, and vitamin D—produce very little change in bone mass and do little to improve bone structure. These agents are a major advance in *preventing* osteoporosis, but to a woman with osteoporotic fractures, they are an *interim* step with little real benefit. Agents that *stimulate* bone formation, and their principles of action, are the subject of the remainder of this chapter.

Until very recently, we were unable even to think about ways to reverse osteoporosis. Now, however, there is reason to be optimistic because we have learned how to add bone to the skeleton by stimulating the cells that form bone without also stimulating the cells that break down bone.

FLUORIDE

Research on fluoride to build bone dates back to the 1960s. Why fluoride? Because a low prevalence of osteoporosis was found in areas with high levels of fluoride in the drinking water. The use of fluoride to treat osteoporosis has waxed and waned in recent years.

Fluoride increases bone mass by stimulating the osteoblast cells to form bone. Fluoride is also incorporated into bone crystal—the part of the bone that gives it strength—so, instead of being composed only of hydroxyapatite, crystal, the bone crystal structure also has fluoride incorporated into it. We know that the addition of fluoride to bone crystal changes some of the properties of bone, but the picture is unclear.

To increase bone mass, we must use agents that increase trabecular bone, cortical bone, or both. Studies reveal that fluoride increases trabecular bone mass in osteoporotic patients—sometimes dramatically. Bone densitometry studies have found increases of about 1 percent *per month* in the lumbar spine. In large studies, there was almost an 8 percent increase in the lumbar spine in 1 year and about a 1 percent increase in the hip over the same period. In general, the fluoride affects trabecular bone. It increases bone mass in the vertebrae—which have a high fraction of trabecular bone—and reduces vertebral fractures. In a 4-year study of women with osteoporotic fractures, those who received 75 milligrams a day of fluoride and supplemental calcium achieved as much as a 35 percent increase in lumbar spine bone mineral density and a 12 percent increase in the femoral neck. Surprisingly, however, the number of new vertebral fractures was *higher* in the fluoride group than in the placebo group. The reason, according to most bone experts, is that the dose of fluoride was too high. This resulted in a decrease in bone strength and thus an increase in the number of fractures in the fluoride-treated group.

When another study was done with a lower dose of a slow-release fluoride preparation (25 milligrams twice a day given over a 14-month cycle—12 months on and 2 months off) for 2.5 years, bone mass increased about 5 percent each year and the number of new vertebral fractures was significantly lower in the fluoride-treated group. So, with fluoride, there is a trade-off—the positive effect of increased bone mass and the negative effect of decreased bone strength. Thus, strict control of the dosage is important to increase the mass of good-quality bone. In general, sodium fluoride in a dose of about 40 milligrams a day can be used to increase bone mass in osteoporotic women with careful monitoring by a physician.

In the United States, sodium fluoride is now available only in very low potency (2- to 5-milligram tablets). (In Europe, by contrast, 10- and 25-milligram tablets are available.) Sodium fluoride frequently causes gastrointestinal irritation. Fluoride can be taken with a calcium supplement. In fact, calcium carbonate acts as an antacid, decreasing the irritating effect of fluoride on the stomach. But fluoride is not well absorbed in the presence of calcium, so the physician must increase the dose of fluoride if the two are taken together.

A new fluoride formulation—slow-release sodium fluoride capsules—has been developed and studied. This type of fluoride is less irritating. In more than 100 patients treated for over 3 years with this slow-release formulation, less than 6 percent had stomach irritation. Studies are continuing, but this form of fluoride is currently not available in the United States.

Early studies found that the abnormal effects on bone mineralization caused by fluoride could be reduced by giving both vitamin D and calcium supplements with the fluoride.

When a woman with osteoporosis is given fluoride, this medication increases her trabecular bone mass over 10 percent after a year or two of treatment. Calcium and vitamin D supplementation together allows the bone to mineralize normally, and this probably prevents further fractures. The amount of bone that fluoride can form is very high. In general, however, bone mass should not increase more than 10 percent a year with this therapy. If it does, this means that a lot of the fluoride is entering the bone crystal, and the bone may become weak and fracture. Therefore, when physicians monitor this bone-building therapy, they check the bone mineral density of the lumbar spine and hip every 6 months. If the increase is more than 5 percent during this period, the fluoride is decreased or stopped for a while. It is common for physicians to prescribe fluoride for 10 months and then nothing for 2 months, after which the cycle is started again.

PARATHYROID HORMONE FRAGMENTS

Parathyroid hormone has many effects on the skeleton and on calcium balance. In fact, a small dose of the hormone by itself can stimulate bone formation. When a small amount of parathyroid hormone is injected into animals or humans, it circulates in the body for only a short time, perhaps as little as 20 minutes. Its major action is to stimulate the bone-forming cells to build bone, although over time there is also an increase in bone resorption. Overall, parathyroid hormone injections seem to produce a positive bone balance—more bone is formed than is resorbed. In osteoporotic animals, daily treatment with an injection of parathyroid hormone fragments—a small part of the parathyroid hormone—returned bone mass to normal in only 4 weeks.

When parathyroid hormone fragments were used in clinical trials with osteoporotic patients, the results were very favorable. One study of osteoporotic women treated with daily parathyroid hormone and vitamin D for 2 years found that trabecular bone mass in the lumbar spine increased about 30 percent, and total spinal bone mass (cortical and trabecular bone) increased 12 percent. But in spite of these gains, there was a small *decrease* in the cortical bone of the forearm compared to the control group.

Since parathyroid hormone treatment increases bone turnover, both formation and resorption, it seems reasonable that if osteoporotic patients were also treated with an agent that blocked resorption, such as estrogen or a bisphosphonate, the bone-forming effects of parathyroid hormone would be greater. And, in fact, this is exactly what happened. When osteoporotic women were treated with antiresorptive agents (estrogen and progesterone) together with parathyroid hormone, bone formation was greater than bone resorption. After 3 years of this combination treatment, spinal trabecular bone mass increased by nearly 13 percent, hip BMD increased by over 3 percent, and no loss of bone mass in the forearm was found.

Currently, many parathyroid hormone fragments are under development for the treatment of osteoporosis. Results of early studies suggest that parathyroid hormone is safe and appears to stimulate bone formation. And unlike fluoride, parathyroid hormone does not become incorporated into the bone crystal, so there is no defect in bone mineralization.

At this time, parathyroid hormone, like insulin, can only be given by a small injection just under the skin. The treatment seems reasonable, but occasionally the calcium level in the blood becomes too high and there is irritation around the injection site. Very few patients have developed antibodies to the parathyroid hormone fragments, which would block the parathyroid hormone from working.

At this time, we can reverse osteoporosis by using an antiresorptive agent, like estrogen or bisphosphonate, together with a bone-forming agent. The two bone-forming agents that are either available or in clinical trials and working their way toward approval by the Food and Drug Administration are slow-release fluoride and parathyroid hormone fragments. While fluoride is available in an easy-to-take tablet, the dose must be kept low so that the bone that is formed is of good quality. Parathyroid hormone fragments appear to stimulate bone formation and, when used with an antiresorptive agent, increase bone mass. Initial studies with parathyroid hormone fragments are very promising, but this compound does require injection. The advantage is that parathyroid hormone is quickly cleared by the body and is not incorporated into the bone; its action is very short-lived. Further work is needed to help physicians and patients decide how to use these bone-building medications most effectively.

GROWTH FACTORS: THE NEW FRONTIER

Growth factors regulate the duplication, differentiation, growth, and function of bone cells. Growth factors are made by several cells in the bone marrow, including osteoblasts, nonosteoblast cells, and other cells. Their job is to regulate osteoblast or nonosteoblast bone cell functions.

There are several regulators of bone formation—parathyroid hormone, insulin, growth hormone, and steroids. All of them probably work by stimulating the production of growth factors, such as insulin-like growth factor (IGF-1), which is made by the osteoblast. Very small, short-term clinical studies involving IGF-1 have been done. In one study of postmenopausal women treated with increasing doses of IGF-1, bone formation increased. Further work is now being done with IGF-1 and other growth factors present in bone that may be used to treat osteoporosis.

SUMMARY

- Current treatments for osteoporosis focus on reducing bone loss by slowing bone breakdown. Today, studies are evaluating bone-building agents that increase bone mass by stimulating bone-forming cells to lay down new bone. Fluoride and parathyroid hormone fragments are two such agents. Both agents increase bone mass in the lumbar spine at a dramatic rate. They also reduce vertebral fractures.

11

Prevention and Treatment of Secondary Osteoporosis

In Chapter 2 we discussed the secondary causes of osteoporosis. Some of them—age, sex, and race; genetic and reproductive factors; and body type, specifically low body mass index—are beyond the person's control. Others—smoking, alcohol use, calcium and vitamin D intake, diet, and drug use—are to some extent individual choices. Let's revisit the conditions in the second category to see what can be done to prevent or treat the bone loss resulting from their incorrect use.

SMOKING AND ALCOHOL USE

As noted in Chapter 2, tobacco may be toxic to bone and may speed up the breakdown of estrogen. Heavy drinking for many years reduces bone mass and speeds up bone loss during menopause and in older men. Like alcohol, it may be directly toxic to bone or may work indirectly through poor nutrition since drinkers substitute alcohol for a healthy, balanced diet. Finally, alcohol interferes with calcium absorption. There is evidence that moderate use of alcohol (e.g., one or two glasses of red wine per day) may actually be beneficial, promoting a healthy heart. But heavy use of any form of alcohol is destructive and should be avoided. By contrast with alcohol, smoking has no redeeming features. This habit should be broken completely.

CALCIUM AND VITAMIN D INTAKE

A diet low in calcium is certain to lead to unhealthy bones, and when such a diet is eaten by older persons—who generally have trouble absorbing calcium—the situation is even more serious. Older women who are not taking HRT are especially at risk because they lack estrogen, which promotes calcium absorption. The best way to build healthy bones before menopause is to eat a balanced diet rich in calcium (see the cookbooks listed in the Appendix) and take at least 1000 milligrams of a calcium supplement. Menopausal women should take 1500 milligrams. Vitamin D supplementation is also important since this vitamin promotes calcium absorption.

DIET

A balanced diet high in vitamins and minerals is essential in childhood, building strong bones and a high peak bone mass in young adults. The diet should be moderate in protein; a high-protein diet, which produces acid and leads to calcium excretion, may increase the risk of osteoporosis. Therefore, a balanced diet that is also high in fruits and vegetables is important. Finally, young women concerned about their appearance should keep in mind the dangers of stringent dieting. This can lead to anorexia nervosa—a state of malnutrition—causing a low peak bone mass in the adult and increasing the risk of bone fractures.

DRUGS

Thyroid Replacement Therapy

Hyperthyroidism and hypothyroidism (see Chapter 2) can both cause bone loss. Hyperthyroidism acts directly; hypothyroidism is controlled by thyroid replacement therapy, too much of which may cause bone loss. In these patients, bone mass must be measured periodically and the dose of the drug adjusted if necessary.

GNRH Agonists

Gonadotropin-releasing hormone (GNRH) agonists are used to treat endometriosis and uterine fibroid tumors in women and prostate tumors in men. These drugs lower estrogen and testosterone levels, leading to bone loss. Patients taking these drugs should consult their physician about ways to prevent this bone loss.

Diuretics

Diuretics, used to control high blood pressure and heart disease, can be either good or bad. Furosemide leads to calcium loss, thiazides to calcium retention. Patients must be aware of the effects of these drugs and compensate for calcium loss accordingly. The physician should be consulted.

Antacids

Antacids are widely used. Those containing aluminum speed up calcium excretion. As with diuretics, patients should be aware of their effects and compensate for the calcium loss accordingly.

Steroids

Steroids are often used to treat acute and chronic inflammatory diseases such as arthritis. But while these medications help to save lives and keep people active, steroid-induced osteoporosis is the most common form of secondary (drug-induced) bone loss.

As we discussed in Chapter 2, steroids create bone loss in several ways. We can now both prevent and treat the disease because we understand how these medications affect bone.

First, steroids cause the body to lose calcium because they prevent it from being absorbed. To prevent calcium loss, all patients on steroids need to take 1500 milligrams of calcium a day in their diet, with supplements, or both. The brands of calcium recommended for postmenopausal osteoporosis are the same as those for steroid osteoporosis. Also, to improve calcium absorption while on steroids, we prescribe vitamin D in the form of two multiple vitamins (800 IU per day).

Steroids lower the levels of gonadal hormones (estrogen in women and testosterone in men), which can also cause bone loss. Therefore, we recommend that postmenopausal women taking steroids consider estrogen replacement therapy. Estrogen not only maintains bone mass in the presence of steroids but also keeps cholesterol low (high cholesterol is a common problem in persons who chronically take steroids). Men on steroids should have their testosterone level checked; if it is low, they should consider testosterone replacement.

Premenopausal women on steroids also have a low estrogen level. These women often report having shorter menstrual periods or lighter bleeding while taking steroids. Because these women lose bone mass due to the low estrogen level, we recommend that they take birth control pills. The pills probably contain enough estrogen to prevent bone loss and keep the cholesterol level low.

Steroids also reduce bone formation, so more bone is resorbed than is formed in each remodeling cycle. Knowing this, it is reasonable to try to reduce bone resorption to prevent steroid-induced bone loss. All of the antiresorptive agents have been used to prevent bone loss in steroid-treated patients. In general, the bisphosphonates prevent bone loss and even provide a gain of about 1 to 2 percent in lumbar spine bone mass within a year of treatment. Studies show that etidronate, alendronate, pamidronate, and residronate prevent bone loss in these patients. Calcitonin has the same good effect. Most of these studies involve patients taking low to medium doses of steroids, such as 5 to 20 milligrams of prednisone a day. We do not know if these medications will prevent bone loss when the doses of steroids are much higher, but we think they will be helpful.

While we can replace calcium and gonadal hormones and give other antiresorptive agents to prevent bone loss, one of the main reason for steroid-induced bone loss is that steroids inhibit bone formation. We are just beginning to study bone-building agents—fluroide and parathyroid hormone fragments—in steroid-induced osteoporotic subjects (see Chapter 10). The results are promising.

The last important reason for treating steroid-induced bone loss is to prevent loss of muscle mass. Steroids break down muscle mass over time, and loss of muscle mass can result in some bone loss, especially cortical (outer envelope) bone. To prevent muscle and cortical bone loss while on steroids, it is important for patients to perform some type of resistance exercise. This exercise can be as simple as swimming twice a week or doing 10 minutes of weight-bearing resistance exercise at home. Patients on steroids should consult their doctor or a physical therapist to obtain the right exercises.

Generally, when we discuss steroid-induced bone loss, we focus on persons who take steroid pills for a long time. Usually infrequent injections of steroids into the muscle or joint, or a few puffs of a steroid inhaler for asthma or other breathing problems, do not cause bone loss. However, use of a steroid inhaler more often than is prescribed, or too many steroid injections into a muscle or joint, allows the steroid level to become higher than normal. Then bone loss will occur.

Understanding how steroids create bone loss and how to prevent this bone loss has been an important breakthrough. Today, with the right medications, we can prevent and perhaps even reverse this disease.

SUMMARY

- Some of the secondary causes of osteoporosis include smoking and alcohol use, low calcium and vitamin D intake, poor diet, and drug use.
- Steroids are the most common cause of drug-induced bone loss. Treatment with calcium and vitamin D supplements and with agents like estrogen, calcitonin, or bisphosphonates can prevent steroid-induced bone loss.
- Muscle-strengthening exercises can maintain muscle mass, which will prevent some steroid-induced bone loss, as well as falls and fractures. Individuals taking steroids should consult their doctor about these options.

MICHELLE: OSTEOPOROSIS FROM STEROIDS USED TO TREAT RHEUMATOID ARTHRITIS

Michelle is 36 years of age, 5 feet 5 inches tall, and weighs 130 pounds. For 10 years, she has suffered from rheumatoid arthritis and has taken a steroid, prednisone, in a dose of 10 milligrams a day, for most of that time. Because of her arthritis pains, she does not exercise. Her calcium intake is about 1000 milligrams a day, and she takes a multiple vitamin that has 400 IU of vitamin D.

Where her bone mineral density was recently measured, it was found to be well below normal for her age.

Prednisone decreases the joint swelling and the pain of arthritis. Unfortunately, it has many side effects, a major one being bone loss. It causes bone loss by inhibiting calcium absorption and increasing calcium loss. It also lowers the estrogen level, which can cause bone loss and decrease bone formation. Taken together, these effects can be serious. Women and men who take more than 5 milligrams a day of prednisone or its equivalent for over 6 months can suffer severe bone loss, which can continue for as long as the medication is used.

The good news for Michelle is that now we understand steroid-induced bone loss and can do several things to prevent further bone loss—even reverse it, if necessary. The first thing Michelle should do is to increase her calcium intake to 1500 milligrams a day, through diet and a supplement, and to increase her vitamin D intake to 800 IU a day to help her absorb the calcium. Next, her doctor should ask Michelle if she is having normal menstrual periods because usually women who take steroids regularly tend to either have very light bleeding or very short menstrual periods. If Michelle has either of these irregularities, the doctor should suggest that she begin to use a birth control pill, which provides some estrogen and will help to build bone mass. If Michelle is already taking a birth control pill or cannot take it, then she should use another medication that prevents bone loss in the presence of steroids—either a bisphosphonate, alendronate, or intranasal calcitonin.

Finally, Michelle should start a low-impact exercise program to build muscle strength. Steroids can cause a loss of muscle mass, but if Michelle can exercise and increase her muscle mass, she can prevent further bone loss.

Michelle may be able to stop taking prednisone at some point, but while she is on it she should probably have another bone mineral density test in about 1 year. This test will tell her doctor if the new medications are working. If she has maintained or gained bone mass since her last measurement, her current therapy should continue. But if she has lost more than 5 to 10 percent of her spinal bone mass during that year, another medication may need to be added to prevent further loss of bone mass.

LISA: STEROID USE AND OSTEOPOROSIS

Lisa is a 65-year-old white woman with a history of rheumatoid arthritis for 20 years. She is 5 feet 3 inches tall and weighs 125 pounds. Recently, she noticed recurrent severe midback pain; an X-ray of her back revealed a new compression fracture. She has taken prednisone in a dose of 10 milligrams a day for her arthritis pain and swelling for about 5 years. She takes ibuprofen and methotrexate (the latter to prevent progression of joint destruction in rheumatoid arthritis) for her arthritis.

Fortunately, Lisa does not have a family history of osteoporosis. Her calcium intake is 1000 milligrams a day, derived from both her diet and a calcium carbonate supplement taken daily along with a multiple vitamin. Three times a week, Lisa participates in an exercise class for arthritis patients. Otherwise, she does no other exercise outdoors and generally stays home because of her painful arthritis.

When Lisa's bone mineral density was measured in the lumbar

spine, it was 0.70 g/cm², with a T score of −3.0. The bone mineral density of her total hip was 0.69 g/cm², with a T score of −2.5.

Lisa has osteoporosis and a painful compression fracture of the spine, probably due to her long use of steroids. It is said that 10 to 20 percent of spinal trabecular bone mass is lost when prednisone is taken in a dose of 7.5 milligrams a day or more. The effects on different individuals vary widely. At any rate, long-term steroid use thins all bones, both cortical and trabecular, and results in a high rate of fractures.

Aside from her steroid use, Lisa's rheumatoid arthritis may also have contributed to her osteoporosis. The inflammation around the joints resulting from the arthritis can cause bone loss, but usually it affects the hands, wrists, ankles, and feet and is less severe in the spine or the hip unless the arthritis is active in those areas. Women who have rheumatoid arthritis have lower bone density than women of the same age who do not. There seems to be no increased risk of osteoporotic fractures in women with arthritis.

A woman who is on steroids for more than a few weeks needs to take 1500 milligrams a day of calcium and 800 IU a day of vitamin D. Lisa will need to increase her calcium intake each day by 500 milligrams, ideally with a supplement of either calcium carbonate or calcium citrate. She can obtain the vitamin D by taking two multiple vitamins a day.

Next, Lisa needs to consider estrogen replacement therapy. Estrogen levels are lowered by steroids, and Lisa's estrogen level is low both from menopause and from steroid use. Steroids cause the cholesterol level to increase. The estrogen therapy can help normalize Lisa's cholesterol level and decrease her risk of heart disease. All of these treatments will prevent Lisa from losing more bone mass while she is on steroids.

Lisa is already doing weight-bearing exercises in her exercise class. This will help to maintain her muscle mass while she is on steroids.

If possible, Lisa should stop taking steroids. If she can do this, some of her lost bone mass will return. After someone has been on steroids a long time, the body becomes dependent on them. If they are stopped quickly, the person can go into shock and may even die. If Lisa wants to try eliminating steroid therapy, she must discuss it with her doctor, since it must be eliminated gradually. Because Lisa has been on steroids for over 10 years, tapering the medication will take a year or more. Luckily, today we have other effective medications for rheumatoid arthritis that usually allow most patients to decrease the dose of steroids to less than 5 milligrams a day.

Lisa will need to have another bone mineral density test after 1 year on these medications. If she has lost more than 5 percent of her hip or spine bone mineral density, then her doctor could consider adding another antiresorptive agent, like calcitonin or a bisphosphonate (alendronate or etidronate) to prevent further loss.

Steroid-induced bone loss is the most common cause of drug-induced osteoporosis, but today it can be both prevented and successfully treated.

MARK: ASTHMA, STEROID TREATMENT, AND THE RISK OF OSTEOPOROSIS

Mark is a 55-year-old white man who suffers from asthma and has been on prednisone for many years. His bone mineral density of the lumbar spine is very low—0.8 g/cm^2, with a T score of −3.0. He has several vertebral compression fractures. Currently, he is 5 feet 9 inches tall and weighs 150 pounds. His usual calcium intake is about 700 milligrams a day, and he walks about five blocks a day for exercise.

It is unusual for men to develop osteoporosis at the age of 55, so a compression fracture in a man younger than 85 indicates another cause of bone thinning. In this case, prednisone is the problem. In a dose greater than 5 milligrams a day taken for 6 months, it causes loss of as much as 20 percent of spinal bone mass. After the initial rapid loss, the bone mass throughout the body declines about 1 to 2 percent a year. Although Mark takes prednisone only 14 days a month, it is enough to have caused bone loss in his spine.

The first thing to do is to increase his daily intake of calcium and vitamin D. Mark must take in 1500 milligrams a day of calcium, either by diet, by supplements, or both. He must also get 800 IU per day of vitamin D to promote calcium absorption. Mark should also have his testosterone level checked. Steroids lower testosterone levels, and testosterone replacement can prevent bone loss. In addition, Mark's physician may decide to start him on antiresorptive therapy—a bisphosphonate or calcitonin—to prevent bone loss in the presence of steroids.

Equally important, Mark should discuss the asthma treatment with his doctor. Many doctors today use steroids that are inhaled instead of taken by mouth. Inhaled steroids work in the lungs and very little enters the blood, so there is almost no effect on bone mass if they are used at the recommended dose. Alternatively, Mark may be able to take an asthma medication other than prednisone.

If Mark can stop taking prednisone, he will regain some of the lost bone mass. We do not know if Mark will regain all of it, but any added bone would help him to prevent new fractures.

MARIAN: ALCOHOLISM AND OSTEOPOROSIS

Marian is a 60-year-old white woman who is 5 feet 7 inches tall and weighs 120 pounds. She has just broken a bone in her foot after walking all day in a shopping mall. Marian entered menopause at age 47 and took estrogen replacement therapy for 2 years but then decided to stop the treatment. She has no family history of osteoporosis. She drinks three or four cups of coffee a day, smokes one or two cigarettes a day, and has been drinking six to eight mixed alcoholic drinks a day for the past 40 years. She developed an ulcer about 5 years ago and takes a medication, called an *H2 blocker*, that decreases her stomach acid. The ulcer has not recurred. Marian's physical activity is limited to walking around the house. Her calcium intake is about 600 milligrams a day from her diet, and she takes a multiple vitamin each day.

Marian's bone mineral density was tested in the femoral neck of her left hip; it measured 0.57 g/cm^2, with a T score of -3.0. The total hip bone mineral density was 0.67 g/cm^2, with a T score of -2.5.

Marian now has osteoporosis. Her main problem is her high consumption of alcohol. By all definitions, Marian is an alcoholic. She is also very thin; this is common since most alcoholics drink their calories and do not eat well. In addition to causing poor nutrition, alcohol depresses bone formation. Both of these conditions lead to low bone mass in young adults. Osteoporosis from alcoholism happens just as often in women as in men.

But Marian's osteoporosis may also result from 11 years of estrogen deficiency as a result of menopause. As noted earlier, she took estrogen replacement for only 2 years, and this therapy must be taken for at least 10 years after menopause to give any protection against osteoporosis.

The major recommendation is for Marian to join a group like Alcoholics Anonymous and to get help with her drinking. Even though her doctor will try to encourage her to take medications to treat the osteoporosis, decreasing her drinking is the most important step she can take to prevent further bone loss.

Since Marian is postmenopausal, she should start to take an anti-resorptive agent to prevent her from losing more bone mass. Estrogen, a bisphosphonate, or calcitonin nasal spray would be appropriate. She will need to increase her daily intake of calcium through a supplement. However, the H2 blocker that she takes minimizes acid production in the stomach. This is important because some calcium supplements, especially calcium carbonate, need stomach acid to help absorption. The calcium supplement that works best for women with low stomach acid is calcium citrate. This is available over the counter, both with and without vitamin D.

Marian should see her doctor again a few weeks after she begins the osteoporosis treatments to have her blood and urine tested for calcium and to see how she is tolerating her medications. Since the doctor will want Marian to use these medications perhaps for many years, Marian should report any side effects that may keep her from taking them regularly. If Marian decides to start estrogen therapy, she should have a baseline mammogram if she has not had one in the last few months, and the mammogram should be repeated every year. Also, since Marian's uterus is intact, she will need to take a progestin for a few days each month or a small dose of a progestin every day to prevent the possibility of uterine cancer.

ANNE: OVERACTIVE THYROID

Anne is a 45-year-old white woman, 5 feet 8 inches tall, weighing about 125 pounds. She has two children. Her mother had osteoporosis and a hip fracture at the age of 70. Anne has a history of an overactive thyroid gland. At the age of 25 she had medical therapy that stopped the thyroid gland from working; since that time, she has been taking thyroid replacement medication. Currently, she is taking Synthroid® in a dose of 0.2 gram a day. Anne eats a regular diet. Her calcium intake is about 1000 milligrams a day, and her vitamin D intake is about 400 IU a day. She works every day and has little time for exercise, so she tries to walk at least one way between work and home, a distance of 2 miles.

When her bone mineral density was measured, the reading was 0.77 g/cm², with a T score of −1.7—a measure well below normal for her age.

Anne's low bone mass is probably the result of a combination of factors—genetics, a history of thyroid disease, and possibly too much thyroid replacement. The thyroid gland is responsible for maintaining the body's metabolic rate. If the body has too little thyroid hormone, the metabolic rate is too low and the person feels cold and tired all the time. By contrast, the person with too much thyroid hormone feels energetic, may have trouble gaining weight, and feels warm or even hot much of the time. Too much thyroid hormone can also increase the bone turnover rate and can cause bone loss and osteoporotic fractures. Recently, we have discovered the level of thyroid hormone that needs to be replaced to prevent bone loss.

First, Anne needs to have her thyroid hormone and thyroid-stimulating hormone levels checked. If the thyroid hormone is too high or the thyroid-stimulating hormone is too low, her thyroid hormone replacement should be reduced. With Anne's family history of osteoporosis and the possibility of too much thyroid hormone, her risk of osteoporosis is high. If her thyroid hormone is lowered to a normal level, her bone mass may stabilize; in fact, it may even increase.

Unfortunately, Anne reached bone maturity with lower than normal bone mass. This may be due to her family history of osteoporosis, and/or the thyroid problem may have resulted in a lot of bone loss over time. At any rate, adjustment of her thyroid medication will prevent her from losing more bone and may even increase it. Over the next 5 years Anne will also probably go through menopause, resulting in further bone loss and increasing her risk of fractures. When Anne does go through menopause, it is critical that she start to take an antiresorptive agent to prevent further bone loss. She will need to discuss the choice with her physician—estrogen, a bisphosphonate, or calcitonin.

Anne's intake of calcium and vitamin D and her exercise are adequate to maintain good bone mass. If her thyroid hormone level is too high and is lowered to normal, Anne may not have trouble gaining a few pounds. As mentioned above, all of her therapy to prevent bone loss will have to be reevaluated when she begins menopause.

JOAN: ANOREXIA NERVOSA

Joan is a 48-year-old white woman, 5 feet 7 inches tall, and weighs 110 pounds. She has two children. Her mother is 68 and has recently had a bone density measurement that is normal. Joan's usual diet contains about 800 milligrams of calcium and 400 IU of vitamin D. She usually exercises once or twice a week, but has noticed that her menstrual periods are no longer coming every month; in fact, she has gone as much as 3 months without a period. She thinks that she is starting to go through menopause and wants to have a bone mineral density measurement done. Her menstrual history is significant for the fact that she did not start menstruating until she was almost 16, and from 18 to 23 years of age, she suffered from anorexia nervosa. During that time, her estrogen levels dropped to that of a postmenopausal woman, and she lost bone. This was a serious problem because Joan had not yet achieved bone maturity, which occurs at around the age of 30 to 35 in most women. Her weight dropped to 85 pounds, and she had no menstrual periods during the 5 years that she was anorexic. At the age of 24, after special counseling, she gained weight and started having regular menstrual periods again.

When Joan's bone mineral density was measured in the lumbar spine, it was found to be 0.74 g/cm^2, and her T score was -2.0. This measurement indicates osteopenia, which means that her bone mass is low. If she loses any more bone mass, she has a moderate risk of fracturing.

Joan's low bone mass reflects the fact that her anorexia nervosa prevented her from achieving peak bone mass, resulting in low adult bone mass. At this point, as Joan is entering menopause, it is critical that she start to take an antiresorptive agent to prevent her from losing bone mass from estrogen deficiency—either estrogen, a bisphosphonate, or calcitonin. Joan also needs to understand the reasons that her bone mass is low at the beginning of menopause and the fact that nutrition is very important to keep her bones healthy during menopause. Joan should increase her calcium intake to 1500 milligrams a day through diet and a supplement and should take 400 to 800 IU of vitamin D a day. Weight-bearing exercise for 30 minutes three or four times a week will also help Joan to maintain strong healthy bones after menopause.

Because Joan has a low bone mass at the beginning of menopause, she should have another bone mineral density test after a year or two to determine if her medications are maintaining her bone mass or if she requires more treatment.

12

Treating the Pains and Problems of Osteoporosis

Pain is one of the most difficult problems associated with osteoporosis. In this chapter, we review some of the breakthroughs and recommendations for treating and managing this pain. Because the osteoporotic fracture is the most severe, or acute, instance of pain, let's consider it first.

THE OSTEOPOROTIC FRACTURE: TREATING ACUTE PAIN

When a woman or a man has an osteoporotic fracture, pain usually develops at the fracture site. The pain may be in the upper back, the lower back, or another area. It can be very sharp or dull and continuous. Usually the muscles around the fractured bone become tense or go into spasm, causing muscle pain. A fracture in the vertebrae of the thorax (the midback or chest area) will usually cause a new pain that feels lodged in the midback, with accompanying painful muscle tension and spasm. This pain increases every time the back is moved—after sitting or lying down or just moving from place to place. Sometimes the back pain will radiate (travel down) the back or around to the abdomen. The pain from a new vertebral fracture can be dull rather than sharp, but it can be chronic (present all the time). Sometimes a woman will see her doctor to find out the reason for the new pain. If an X-ray is taken a compression fracture of the vertebrae may be revealed. But in the first few days to weeks after the fracture, the X-ray may show nothing. On examination, typically there will be a painful spot in the back area where the vertebral fracture has occurred. Also, around the fracture, the muscles next to the spine will be very tense and painful to the touch. This pain can last for periods ranging from a few weeks to 2 months; then slowly it resolves. If the doctor is not sure of the cause of the back pain, he or she may order a special X-ray or a bone scan. For a bone scan, a radioactive substance is injected into the bloodstream and circulates to areas of active inflammation, which are common around an area of fractured bone. The bone scan will show fractured vertebrae long before a regular X-ray.

Medical Treatment

The acute pain of an osteoporotic fracture may need medical treatment, depending on how severe it is. For example, mild pain, noticed by the patient only once or twice a day, or pain that is dull and nagging but not severe, can usually be treated with a simple analgesic (pain killer) like Tylenol® (325 milligrams). The patient can take up to 10 tablets a day safely. This medication can also be taken every 4 to 6 hours during the day and night as needed.

If the pain becomes stronger, waking the patient at night, or is so bothersome that the patient cannot perform day-to-day activities, then a stronger pain medication is needed. The next type of medication to try is a nonsteroidal anti-inflammatory drug (NSAID). NSAIDs are commonly used for all types of pain and include ibuprofen (Motrin® or Advil®), naprosyn (Aleve®, Naprosyn®, or Naprolan®), piroxicam (Feldene®), etodolac (Lodene®), sulindac (Clinoril®), and diclofenac (Voltaren®). Some of them can be obtained over the counter in low doses, but in higher doses they require a doctor's prescription. NSAIDs can help decrease the pain and muscle spasm of a new vertebral fracture and can be taken once or twice a day as needed. They should be taken with food to avoid gastric or stomach irritation.

In some women with an acute vertebral compression fracture, simple analgesics or NSAIDs are not helpful and stronger pain medications are needed for a short period of time. Sometimes doctors prescribe narcotic analgesics including medications with codeine, meperidine, tramadol, or percodan. These medications relieve some of the acute, sharp pain from a compression fracture, but they also cause undesirable side effects, including nausea, drowsiness, and constipation. Constipation can be a serious problem because when a woman has to strain to have a bowel movement, the back pain from her fracture increases. Therefore, stronger narcotic medications, although very effective, should be used sparingly to avoid making the situation worse. Another medication that can help reduce the pain from an acute fracture is calcitonin. This is usually given by injections of 50 to 100 IU per day for 1 to 2 weeks, then is gradually reduced and stopped after 4 to 6 weeks. Calcitonin, like the narcotic medications, should be used only after simple analgesics or NSAIDs are found to be ineffective.

Fortunately, the acute back pain from a new fracture usually dissipates over 3 to 4 weeks. Sometimes, when the pain is very severe, a doctor may order complete bed rest on a hard mattress with a soft covering, like sheepskin or a 2-inch foam pad. During bed rest, it is important to have a pillow under the head and one under the knees to avoid straining the spine. Sometimes it is more comfortable for the patient to lie on the side rather than on the back. When lying on the side, the knees should be bent a bit, which usually makes the pain more tolerable.

Heating Pads and Massage

A heating pad or a gentle massage of the muscles around the fractured vertebrae can also help to decrease the pain of muscle spasms. Heat administered for about 20 to 30 minutes, using either a heating pad or an infrared light, may be helpful. If an infrared heat lamp is used, it must be kept about 2 feet from the back to prevent burning of the skin. Massage can be done by gentle stroking. Deep massage should be avoided since heavy pressure can increase the pain in the first few weeks after a fracture.

Back Supports

If the acute back pain from a fracture continues despite a few days of bed rest, heat treatments, and analgesic medications, a back support can be used when the patient needs to walk. Usually a soft back support can be found in a pharmacy, drugstore, or medical supply store. It supports the patient with acute back pain when she needs to be up and walking about.

Rigid (hard) back supports can also be used to reduce the acute pain of a fracture, but they are not very well tolerated by elderly women because they are very tight and confining and may weigh up to 4 pounds, causing additional discomfort. Sometimes a semirigid back support will be prescribed for acute back pain from an osteoporotic fracture. This is a reasonable alternative because it has shoulder straps that help spread the strain throughout the skeleton. If a back brace is used with acute pain, it must be used only for a short time—no longer than 2 to 3 weeks—because it causes atrophy (wasting) of the abdominal muscles that support the spine, resulting in chronic back pain and loss of muscle strength. The use of a back support should be discussed with the physician, who will present the benefits and risks of the brace and provide proper instructions on how to get the most out of it. A back brace must usually be obtained from a physical therapist, an occupational therapist, or a special orthopedic store. The physician's office can help the patient get this information.

THE OSTEOPOROTIC FRACTURE: TREATING CHRONIC PAIN

Chronic pain after an osteoporotic fracture may result from the fracture itself or from a new curvature of the spine—called *kyphosis* or *scoliosis*—which is caused by overstretching of the ligaments of the spine. As we age, changes occur in the spine even without osteoporotic fractures. For example, the intervertebral disk—soft cushioning material between the bones or vertebrae that give the spine its shock-absorbing ability—shrink with age, becoming stiffer and less compliant. As spinal flexibility decreases, other changes may add to the difficulties—weakened muscles, poor or weak back extensors, and the added effect of gravity. The daily strain of physical activities can often result in a kyphotic posture—a bending forward of the upper back in elderly women and men even without osteoporosis. Kyphosis can be mild to severe, depending on the number of vertebral fractures and the other changes in the spine as the person ages. In women with severe kyphosis, the pressure on the lower part of the rib cage over the rim of the pelvis can cause pain and tenderness in the pelvic area. This pain occurs because the lower ribs are pressed into the pelvic bone. Severe kyphosis also causes loss of height, which can increase the pain.

Chronic pain—intermittent pain that is a daily remainder of the disease—is a major problem and is difficult to manage. Although the causes of chronic pain are not well understood, the problems it creates are many. Persons with chronic back pain do not like to stand up for long because this usually increases the pain. And since the back muscles that support the spine are not used much, they weaken, creating worse posture and more pain. When muscles are not used very much, they weaken and persons are limited by what they can then do physically.

Persons with chronic pain avoid movement and begin to limit their activities. Eventually, the pain limits their ability to perform simple daily activities. And although pain may not be the primary reason for lower self-esteem or depression, it can definitely add to these problems. Those with chronic pain are more likely to lose their social roles and need social support.

Persons with chronic pain from osteoporosis may also require an analgesic for pain relief. These pain medications work only for a short time. Chronic or continued use of strong pain medications can lead to drug addition.

Exercise

The only way to treat the chronic pain from compression fractures and the associated changes in posture or kyphosis is through measures that improve the posture and bring the spine more upright. Some improvements in posture may occur with exercise if back extension exercises (which stretch the muscles next to the spine) are included. Sometimes the application of heat, either using an infrared lamp or a heating pad before beginning exercise, makes the exercise program more tolerable. Taking an analgesic before exercising is also helpful. Sometimes, when the kyphosis is severe, the person may experience pain and have difficulty taking a deep breath. In such cases, a wheelchair may be needed.

Strengthening exercises, properly done, can improve the muscles that support the upper and lower spine and can be an important part of therapy. Back extension exercises improve back strength and reduce pain. They can be done in a chair or lying on the stomach. A sitting position may be best because it avoids or minimizes pain in persons with severe osteoporosis.

In a sitting position (Figure 12.1), the person holds the back straight and the elbows at a 90-degree angle, then stretches them back and tries to touch the elbows together from behind. If a back extension exercise is done while lying on the stomach, a towel or pillow should be placed under the abdomen while lying down to make the exercise more comfortable. The person then lifts the head away from the floor about 15 degrees (1 or 2 inches).

Back extension exercises, done regularly, prevent the spine from becoming more kyphotic. Initially, the person should perform these exercises for a few minutes twice a day, working up to at least 5 minutes at each session. If he or she can do them routinely, further changes in posture will be prevented (Figure 12.2).

Many persons with osteoporosis and back pain may not realize that

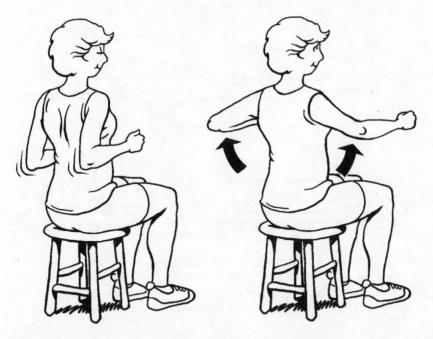

Figure 12.1 *A back extension exercise. Back extension exercises can be done in a sitting position. Sitting avoids or decreases pain in patients who have severe osteoporosis or who have recently had a new vertebral compression fracture. These exercises should be done for 5–10 minutes three times a week and increased as tolerated.*

they have weak abdominal muscles. Therefore, the most successful exercise regimens for these women include both extension exercises for the spine and isometric (muscle-strengthening) exercises for the abdomen (Figures 12.3, 12.4, and 12.5). Together these exercises improve the muscular support of the spine, but they need to be done with supervision or very carefully so that they do not cause undue ligament strain or injury. For example, the person must lie on the back with the hands at the side next to the pelvis and lift the legs about 15 to 20 degrees. When this exercise is repeated for 5 to 10 minutes twice a day, the abdominal muscles will begin to strengthen. Another way to strengthen the abdominal muscles is by lying flat, with the hands at the sides and the knees bent at a 15- to 20-degree angle. Lift the head and try to touch the head to the chest. This exercise, done for 5 to 10 minutes twice a day, will begin to strengthen the abdominal muscles.

The exercise program must be tailored to each person, depending on a number of factors—his or her overall physical condition, age,

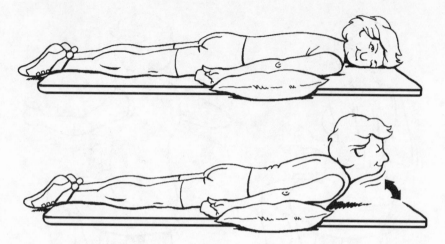

Figure 12.2 *Another back extension exercise. Back extension exercises can also be done while lying on the abdomen. This exercise is done by lifting the head and chest for a few seconds at a time. A floor pad and a pillow should be used for support. This exercise should be done 5–10 times, three times a week, and increased as tolerated.*

and the severity of the osteoporosis. Initially, it may be easier to begin by working on back extension exercises first. These can be done in a chair until more strength and balance develop. There is no magic bullet for the treatment of chronic pain and the problems that occur in a woman's skeleton after osteoporotic fractures. But exercises, if done properly, can be safe and effective in strengthening the muscles around the spine.

Extensor Versus Flexor Exercise

While extensor exercises of the spine—those that make the person lean the head back—help prevent forward curvature of the spine, flexion exercises—those that make the body lean forward—do not (Figure 12.6). Flexion exercises increase compression forces on the spine, further increasing the chance of developing an anterior wedge fracture. A study was done to determine the effect of back extension and flexion exercises on women with established postmenopausal osteoporosis, and the patients were followed up for 1 to 6 years. All of those who performed back flexion exercises developed new vertebral compression fractures compared to only 20 percent of those who performed back extension exercises. In the group that performed both types of exercise, about 50 percent developed new vertebral compression fractures. Further, in the group that did flexion exercises,

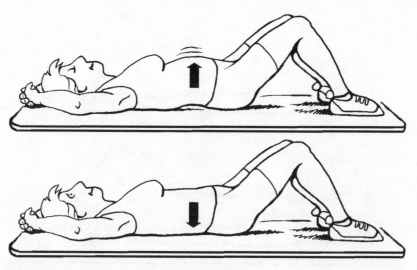

Figure 12.3 *An exercise to strengthen the abdominal muscles. This isometric exercise is easily done at home. It decreases lumbar lordosis by pulling up the abdomen. It is best to lay on a floor mat and, with the knees bent 90 degrees, to press the small of the lower back into the mat. This exercise helps to strengthen abdominal muscles and lumbar flexing muscles. At first, this exercise should be done slowly, 5–10 times in one sitting once or twice a week, increasing it to once a day.*

anterior wedge fractures occurred more often. The authors naturally concluded that flexion exercises are harmful. Most physicians and physical therapists recommend back extension exercises for patients with postmenopausal osteoporosis.

Weight-Bearing Activities

We learned in Chapter 9 that exercise that stresses the body can contribute to skeletal health. Persons with osteoporosis should walk and climb stairs when possible or use a stair-climbing exerciser, if they can tolerate it, to exercise in order to maintain their bone mineral density. If a person with an osteoporotic fracture stops walking and other weight-bearing activities, he or she will lose both muscle mass and bone mass, further weakening the bones and balance and increasing the risk of falling, which can result in a hip fracture.

We know that weight-bearing exercise stresses the lower extremities and promotes bone health. However, stressing the upper extremities with exercises that expose the spine to high compressive forces can be too much for the osteoporotic spine. Exercises involving the

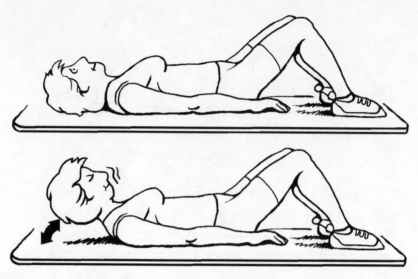

Figure 12.4 *Another exercise to strengthen abdominal muscles. It is best to lay on the back and lift the knees about 45 degrees. Then lift the head toward the chest. This exercise helps to strengthen the abdominal muscles and prevents kyphosis from worsening. At first, this exercise should be done slowly, 5–10 times in one sitting once or twice a week, increasing it to once a day.*

upper extremities must be used only when the proper techniques and limits have been established by a trained health or exercise professional. Other types of exercise can be helpful without risking injury. The elastic band is a safe exercise device that strengthens the back extensor muscles and those around the shoulder girdle that promote good posture. Large, durable elastic bands provide enough resistance for strengthening of back muscles (Figure 12.7). Place an elastic band about 2 feet long over a bar about 2 feet above your head. When you grasp either end of the band and pull down, the latissimus dorsi and shoulder adductors (upper back muscles) are strengthened. The elastic band can also be used by holding either end with one hand and standing with both feet on the middle of the band. When you pull the band backward, the shoulder adductors and extensors get a workout. When you pull your arms up over your head, the back extensor muscles are strengthened.

If a person with osteoporosis wants to do low to moderate muscle-strengthening and weight-loading exercises that may decrease bone loss in the upper extremities and upper spine, he or she may do very gentle weight lifting (Figure 12.8). The maximum weight for each hand should usually be 1 to 3 pounds and should never exceed 5

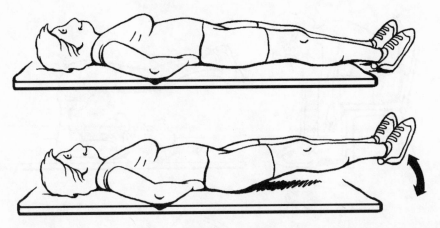

Figure 12.5 *Another exercise to strengthen the abdominal muscles. This exercise is done by lying on the back and placing the hands in the space between the spine and the mat. Then lift the legs, one at a time, about 20 to 40 degrees above the pad for a few seconds and lower them to the mat. At first, this exercise should be done slowly, 5–10 times in one sitting once or twice a week, increasing it to once a day.*

pounds. The amount of weight lifted needs to be prescribed according to the person's bone mass, the severity of her osteoporosis, and the condition of the muscles of her upper extremities. Weight lifting can be performed in a sitting position by persons who have poor or unsteady balance or arthritis of the lower extremities. The shoulder extensors can be strengthened by lifting the weights and putting the shoulder joint through its full range of motion.

Back Supports

Back supports, or braces, can be used by persons in chronic pain stemming from osteoporosis or fractures. The back support can correct posture. Usually semirigid or rigid back supports are used, depending on the severity of the spinal osteoporosis, the patient's tolerance of the brace, and the length of time since the osteoporotic fracture. Back supports correct posture by reminding the patient to avoid heavy lifting or bending while doing daily activities. Since the brace prevents the patient from increasing forward-bending posture, the compressive forces on the spine are minimized. The back support may be used to correct posture and can be added to other measures used to manage pain—for example, simple pain medications and physical therapy.

Unfortunately, as noted earlier, continued use of a back support

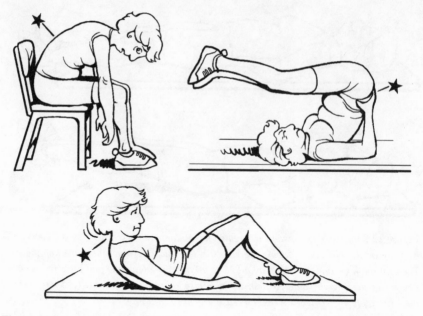

Figure 12.6 *Exercises to be avoided by women with osteoporosis, especially with vertebral fractures. These exercises flex the lumbar spine, increasing thoracic kyphosis and forward flexion.*

will result in weak abdominal muscles, and back extensor muscles may grow even weaker. Therefore, a back support can help a person with severe pain walk and do some other activities, but it must be used with caution and for very short periods of time, or the benefits will be outweighed by the problems. Generally it is best to use physical therapy and an exercise program while wearing the back support to try to prevent muscle atrophy.

PREVENTING FALLS

The dreaded event in osteoporosis is a fracture. In an elderly person with osteoporosis, fractures may become common, but osteoporosis is not the only cause of age-related fractures. Osteoporotic fractures are generally associated with a specific episode of trauma, usually a fall. In the elderly, poor vision, muscle weakness, poor coordination, and poor posture all contribute to a fall. Devices like canes or walkers can improve an elderly person's gait or walk and prevent falls.

There is a whole range of gait-assisting devices—from simple canes, to supportive canes with a broader base of support, to those with prongs, including walkers and wheeled walkers. If a woman has

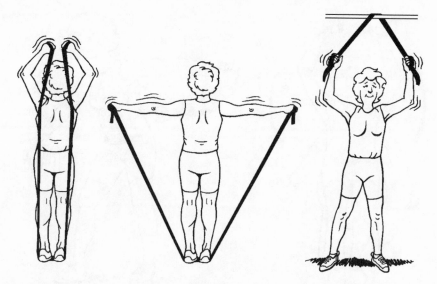

Figure 12.7 *Exercises with an elastic band. These exercises strengthen shoulder and back extensor muscles. Strengthening these muscles can prevent a kyphotic posture.*

pain only on one side of her lower back that radiates to her buttocks and hip, the use of a cane on the side opposite the painful one can decrease the pain of walking. Canes increase the base of support, improving the patient's balance. Walkers, if wheeled, eliminate some of the strain on the osteoporotic spine that would otherwise result from lifting the walker. In general, walkers are more supportive than canes and are used for limited walking activities.

Physical or occupational therapists are the appropriate medical professionals to consult regarding assistive devices. The best way to figure out which device is best is to decide what feels comfortable and what activities you still wish to perform. This information allows the therapist to decide which type of assistive device you need. Usually a physical or occupational therapist in your community will have these devices. You may want to ask your physician to refer you to one of these health care professionals.

THE QUALITY OF LIFE AFTER AN OSTEOPOROTIC FRACTURE

The detection, prevention, and treatment of osteoporosis have increased greatly in recent years. However, we do not yet have a cure for this disabling disease. And because osteoporosis is a serious

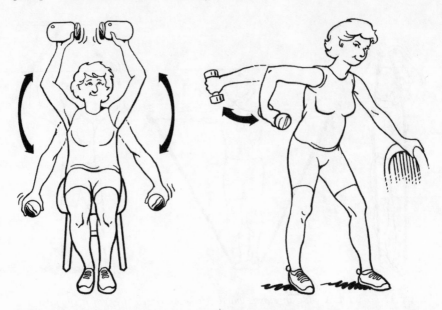

Figure 12.8 *Exercises to strengthen the shoulder extensor muscles. Strengthening these muscles can prevent a kyphotic posture. For this exercise, either use a can of soup or purchase 1- to 3-pound free weights; do not hold more than 5 pounds in each hand. Lift the weights from the side up over the head. Bend the knees slightly to avoid straining the lumbar spine. The person who is unable to lift the arms above the head can put the hands with weights together at the chest and then extend the arms fully. Keep one hand on the chair to maintain balance if you perform the exercise standing up. It is important to put one hand on the back of a chair for balance and to bend one knee to maintain balance.*

worldwide problem, we must focus not only on prevention and treatment but also on ways to deal with the results of the disease, like pain, depression, and loss of self-esteem. For patients with osteoporosis, quality-of-life issues are very important.

Helplessness and Depression

Unfortunately, very little work has been done on the ways in which osteoporosis affects psychological and social well-being. Much of the information we have comes from conversations with patients. As with any chronic disease, patients with osteoporosis can become depressed. People with osteoporosis often feel hopeless in the face of a disease that seems to have taken over their bodies. This reaction occurs most often when a nontraumatic event like a simple cough results in a vertebral compression fracture or when a fall during normal daily activity causes a fracture that immobilizes the person, reinforcing her feeling of helplessness. No matter how the fracture occurs, patients begin to wonder about the quality of life in their remaining years, and they begin to fear that they will experience more fractures during their daily activities. This fear of fracturing often limits their activities, which can reduce overall physical fitness and often leads to more falls. Also, when they limit their daily activities, patients can become less active and less social. All of these changes can make depression worse.

Chronic pain in an elderly person can result in feelings of helplessness and hopelessness, and the longer it goes on, the more hopeless the person may feel. Chronic pain takes up a great deal of emotional energy, leaving very little to manage one's life. Indeed, it is the chronic pain of osteoporosis that makes this disease so hard to treat. Persons with chronic pain from osteoporosis report that they wake up during the night because the pain is so great and feel exhausted the following day. Depression becomes a problem when these persons begin to picture the rest of their lives as filled with pain.

Depression from osteoporosis takes many different forms. Some persons have trouble sleeping, lose their appetite, lose interest in their normal activities, and may withdraw from friends and family. Also, patients with many osteoporotic fractures, who experience severe functional limitations and changes in their appearance, may look on death as a relief from their suffering and pain.

Anxiety

Anxiety too is often experienced by persons with multiple vertebral or hip fractures. The frailty and chronic pain that are part of many of their lives increase their tension and worry. Some persons become obsessed with the treatment of their disease, fearing the worst. Others experience more stress because they expect more of themselves than is possible now that they have osteoporosis. For example, women who are no longer able to clean their house report that they feel stress.

Interference with Physical and Social Activities

These women may also be unable to socialize, which can frustrate them as well. And as their physical appearance changes, their self-esteem diminishes and they may avoid social obligations due to embarrassment.

A single vertebral compression fracture or low bone mineral density does not in itself lead to diminished self-esteem or a feeling of despair. But over time, vertebral compression fractures prevent persons from doing their usual tasks and can reduce their self-esteem because they feel they can no longer make a contribution. When persons with established osteoporosis no longer enjoy their hobbies and do not work inside or outside of their homes, they are at risk for depression. Persons who were active and productive before developing osteoporosis find this condition especially difficult and suffer emotionally.

These psychological problems usually begin slowly. When a loss of height is small at the beginning of the disease, it can be easily ignored. But as it progresses and a kyphotic posture is assumed, a woman especially may see herself as deformed and unfamiliar to herself. As the disease progresses, a woman's shape changes. Her rib cage is much closer to her pelvis than when she was younger, and her clothes no longer fit. When she goes shopping, its difficult to find any clothes that fit her new shape.

There are also social consequences of osteoporosis. Most women and men assume many roles—spouse, parent, worker, friend, church or hospital volunteer. Most healthy adults participate in social groups, and when a chronic disease occurs, they cannot fulfill their commitments. Depending on its severity, osteoporosis may force them to give up some or all of their responsibilities. Jobs that require lifting, twisting, carrying, or bending can no longer be done. On the other hand, sedentary jobs are also discouraged because they add to the muscle weakness due to the disease. With the loss of a job, persons experience many problems related to self-esteem and a sense of self-worth. Financial concerns also become an issue.

The person's role within the family can also change. A grandfather who likes to carry his grandchildren around can no longer do so safely with osteoporosis. This will deny him some of the bonding that can occur between grandfathers and grandchildren. Women who cook and clean the house for their husbands and other family members will no longer get satisfaction from these tasks and sometimes must hire someone to do these chores.

Some Solutions

Serious as these problems are, there are ways to cope. Occupational therapists offer devices that allow persons to reach farther than is physically possible. Other devices can help them prepare meals and shop or fold the laundry. The best thing that an occupational therapist can do is to work with clients to find out what their limitations are and develop strategies to allow them to perform their tasks with the help of assistive devices. The therapist can also teach them how to modify their habits to accommodate the new physical limitations.

Depression, anxiety, and a host of other emotions can seem overwhelming at times, but there are a few simple guidelines that may offer help. As with chronic disease, altered appearance can be a severe blow. Unfortunately, doctors are often not trained to take care of these special needs, nor do they have the time to help patients develop strategies to compensate for these changes. One of the most successful sources of help is the local osteoporosis support group, where patients can learn from others how best to cope with their new challenges. Other support groups, such as the local arthritis foundation, are also there to provide help at each stage of the disease.

However, persons with chronic pain should be prescribed some pain relief medication to prevent the depression, helplessness, and fatigue associated with this condition. It is important to start with simple pain killers like aspirin and anti-inflammatory drugs and then progress to stronger pain killers such as Tylenol® with codeine or Percoset®. In general, very short-acting pain relievers and antianxiety medications are safe. Pain relievers must be prescribed carefully because many of them cause drowsiness in the elderly, which can result in falls and accidents. Therefore, these medications should be used only after a careful explanation is given to the patient and caregivers. The treatment of chronic pain in osteoporosis should start with very low doses of the medication and should be increased very slowly.

SUMMARY

- Osteoporotic fractures cause acute and then chronic pain. Pain control is essential to keep osteoporotic patients comfortable and active and to prevent depression.
- Acute pain can be treated with medication (mild pain killer, NSAID, or narcotic analgesic, either alone or in combination), heating pads, massage, and back support.
- Treatment of chronic pain includes strengthening back extensor muscles with exercise and weight-bearing activities such as walking that improve balance and strengthen back support.

- Gait-assisting devices, including canes and walkers, can prevent the osteoporotic patient from falling.
- Patients with osteoporotic fractures may feel anxious, helpless, and depressed due to lifestyle limitations and changes in appearance. Physical devices are now available to help them function independently at home. Therapists can teach new ways of working, and support groups bring patients together and provide information.

MARTHA: TREATING THE ACHES AND PAINS OF OSTEOPOROSIS

Martha would be a typical 78-year-old grandmother if it weren't for her history of osteoporosis. She has had five vertebral compression fractures, lost 3 inches in height, has a kyphotic posture, and suffers from chronic back pain. Her physician gave her medications to prevent further bone loss, including calcium supplements of 1500 milligrams a day, a daily multiple vitamin, and alendronate. Martha is now interested in treatments to control her chronic back pain.

Because of her vertebral fractures, Martha usually has chronic back pain. In contrast to the pain of a new fracture, caused by bone and muscle spasm, chronic back pain from compression fractures is the result of mechanical strain and overloading of the back's extensor muscles in reaction to the forward bending of the fractured segment of the spine. The tightness of the muscles that support and surround the spine—the *paraspinal* and *anterior thoracic muscles*—may also ache because they too are reacting to the forward tipping of the spine. The chronic tightness of these muscles may cause pain and limit movement of the spine, the rib cage, and the shoulders. And if these muscles around the spine are weak, continued strain on them can contribute to the chronic pain.

Martha says that her pain usually is dull and achy, but at times it can also be sharp, like a pin prick. The pain becomes noticeable when she is doing daily chores around the house during the day, like cooking and bending over to remove clothes from the washing machine. She also notices the pain when she has been sitting for over 15 to 20 minutes.

Martha's pain may be due to irritation of the spinal nerves caused by forward angulation of the spine, which causes the nerves to travel outside the spine to reach their destination. Occasionally, the sharp pain that Martha feels is from a spinal nerve that is being pinched or irritated, much like the pain caused by a slipped disk.

Martha's treatment should be aimed at controlling her back pain, but this pain has many different causes, including muscle weakness, muscle tightness, nerve pain, and poor posture. The best way to start is to have Martha see a physical therapist, who can help her first by improving her posture and later, hopefully, by reducing her future risk of fractures. The therapist will instruct Martha to do specific exercises that will stretch her back muscles, strengthen her back extensor and abdominal muscles, and improve her posture. By strengthening the muscles that support the spine—the back extensor, abdominal, and pelvic muscles—Martha will gain the support needed to perform her daily activities. Examples of the exercises that the physical therapist may teach her are presented in this chapter.

The physical therapist can also show Martha ways to support her back when she is sitting and doing these exercises so that she can prevent pain before it starts. Cushions that fit in a chair and are hollowed out, so that Martha's back can be supported while she is sitting, can be obtained from specialty stores. If she cannot obtain a cushion, then a pillow or a rolled-up towel can be used to support the small of her back. These cushioning devices allow the muscles around the back to relax while Martha is sitting. At the same time, they provide good alignment or support for the spine, avoiding flexion that can make the posture worse.

Ice or heat can also help decrease muscle spasms and tightness. Other methods—electric stimulation, ultrasound, or massage—may be very helpful in relieving or controlling pain. Some of these methods may be useful at the beginning of an exercise program when the muscles are weak and are being used in a different, more demanding way. But it is important to keep in mind that while ice, heat, massage, electrical stimulation, or ultrasound can help relieve some of the pain, none of these methods alone is effective in controlling pain completely and restoring Martha's ability to function. They must be used in conjunction with a medication and an appropriate exercise program.

Sometimes, when the pain is very bad and Martha cannot even walk around the house, she can use a soft elastic low back support. This can help her until her exercises strengthen her postural muscles and relieve her pain. She should not use the back support for pain relief on a regular basis because it can cause muscle atrophy, leading to less motion of the spine and increasing her risk of another fracture.

Unfortunately, Martha's stooped posture is permanent. Nothing can be done to reverse the vertebral compression fractures that she has already suffered. But there is much that Martha can do. Her physician and physical therapist have encouraged her to participate regularly in an exercise program that will keep her postural muscles strong and prevent further bending of the spine. The exercises will also prevent her head and shoulders from being pushed forward. Although it will never be as easy as it once was, Martha must stay as active as possible to prevent her muscles from getting weaker and her bones from becoming thinner, as well as to prevent her from becoming depressed. If she withdraws, she will not get exercise and will only become more depressed.

With the help of illustrations, Martha can see how she can begin to move her body in order to remain active. Once she understands her limitations and the proper ways to move, she can stop worrying about an injury and feel motivated to join a regular exercise program. She can also do simple things in her own home to help her prevent injury and falls. For example, when she gets out of bed, rises from a chair, puts on her clothes, cleans the house, or removes clothes from the washing machine, she should bend her hips and knees and keep her spine in a neutral position. She should also avoid any activities that make her flex or bend her spine forward. These include picking things up from the floor, lifting heavy bags of groceries, or lifting grandchildren.

The best weight-bearing activities for Martha do not require bending, lifting, or twisting. They include walking, slow aerobic exercise, and dancing. Other activities, like swimming, or bicycling, are helpful for muscle strengthening and coordination as well as cardiovascular fitness, but they do not improve muscle mass. Unless activities load the skeleton by adding stress to the bones that exceeds the normal stress level for daily activities, no bone building will take place in patients with osteoporosis.

Martha returns to her doctor for a checkup 3 months after her initial visit. She has been taking Tylenol® as needed for pain—usually two or three times a day—and doing exercises to improve her posture twice a day, each session lasting about 15 minutes. She feels very good about things and rates her pain as 3 out of 10 (where 1 is low and 10 is high). She asks her doctor how long she needs to keep doing the exercises.

Any doctor or health care provider would be happy with Martha's good news. Her pain is reduced, she has learned how to work with her disability, and she is less depressed. But her question shows that the reality of her situation hasn't sunk in. Martha must exercise for the rest of her life. The benefits of exercise will last only as long as the exercise program continues. Martha should plan to see her physical therapist about every 6 months to review her exercises and to solve problems as they come up. With new challenges, Martha's exercise routine may need to be changed.

ELSA: PREVENTING FALLS AT HOME

Elsa is an 83-year-old woman who recently missed a step in her house and fell, fracturing her hip. She lives alone, so she had to push herself along the floor until she reached the telephone to call her daughter, who came right over and called an ambulance to take Elsa to the hospital. The doctors at the hospital repaired the fracture surgically, and Elsa entered a rehabilitation program at the hospital, which turned out well. Upon discharge, Elsa and her daughter decided that it would be safer for Elsa to move in with her daughter. Elsa now walks with a cane and, understandably, is afraid of falling again. She asks her doctor what she and her daughter can do to prevent another fall.

Elsa's concern about falling is real; one hip fracture creates a very high risk of having another. The first thing that Elsa needs is treatment to prevent her from losing any more bone. Her doctor took a brief dietary history and found that Elsa's usual daily calcium intake is about 500 milligrams, so he recommended a supplement of calcium carbonate—1000 milligrams a day—along with a multiple vitamin so that she obtains enough vitamin D to absorb the calcium. Elsa also needed a medication to prevent further bone loss. Her doctor started her on alendronate at a dose of 10 milligrams a day. This medication not only prevents bone loss but also creates some new bone at the hip and spine after a few years.

Once medical therapy was worked out, Elsa needed a rehabilitation program to help her walk again. A thorough evaluation was needed to determine what factors increased her risk of falling and fracturing her hip again. Such factors in elderly women include poor vision or poor depth perception, use of medications that may affect vision and reflexes, dizziness and poor balance, recent weight loss, and problems with moving around or walking. Elsa's doctor checked her vision, balance, and motor coordination and reviewed her medications to be sure that she was not taking anything that would create problems with walking or keeping her balance.

A visiting nurse inspected Elsa's daughter's house, looking for places that might cause problems for Elsa. Several conditions can be dangerous—a slippery kitchen floor, a badly positioned handrail (or no handrail), loose steps or stones on a patio or driveway, a toilet seat without handrails, or a deep bathtub that is difficult to get out of. This review of Elsa's daughter's home resulted in certain modifications that helped alleviate Elsa's fears and may prevent her from falling again.

ALICE: THE FULL TREATMENT AFTER A HIP FRACTURE

Alice is a 75-year-old woman who has just suffered a right hip fracture when she tripped on a shoe in the hall of her house. She was taken to the hospital and had surgery for the fracture that same day. She weighs 120 pounds and is 5 feet 4 inches tall. She has shrunk 2 ½ inches since the age of 25 and thinks that this happened in the past 5 years. Her mother died young, but she remembers that her father's sister had osteoporosis when she was in her 70s. Alice started menopause at the age of 51 and did not take estrogen replacement therapy. Today her calcium intake from her diet is about 700 milligrams a day. She walks around her house but does not get any exercise. In fact, she sits watching television or playing cards most of the day. A bone mineral density scan of her left hip produced a reading was 0.62 g/cm^2, with a T score of $-$ 2.7.

Unfortunately, often the first sign of osteoporosis in elderly women is a hip fracture. And with the fracture comes many problems. For example, a small percentage of women who suffer hip fractures die during or shortly after the surgery because of the stress of the surgery and their poor general health. There is also a recovery period after a hip fracture, and since it can be hard for patients to get around on their own, they may need to live in a nursing home or an extended care facility for a while. This separates people from their personal belongings, as well as their family and friends, which can be painful. A few elderly women who suffer a hip fracture never live independently again. So a hip fracture, the end result of osteoporosis, can be a turning point in a woman's life. The fracture can change her from an independent to a dependent person.

There are many things to do when a woman has a hip fracture. Although she will need calcium and antiresorptive agents to prevent her from losing more bone, there are also other risk factors that can be modified to prevent further fractures. These factors include a sedentary lifestyle, use of medications that cause drowsiness or sedation, poor balance, and poor depth perception. These modifiable risk factors are the ones that a woman like Alice needs to work on. For example, Alice's doctor will find out how many hours Alice spends sitting down during the day to determine her activity levels, find out what her current weight is and if it has changed recently, and what medications she takes. Her doctor will also refer her to an ophthalmologist to find out how accurate her depth perception is and, if necessary, prescribe new eyeglasses. These modifiable risk factors have only recently been identified, and it is too early to know from ongoing studies if modifying some or all of them will decrease the risk of hip fractures. Still, if Alice has lost weight recently, or if she is below the recommended weight for her height, efforts should be made to increase her daily calorie intake with foods that she enjoys to increase her weight. Next, her doctor will check her balance by having her walk along a straight line in the office (like a sobriety test) to see if she can maintain it. If Alice has problems, she should see both a physical therapist to learn exercises that can improve her balance and an occupational therapist to obtain a cane, a walker, or another assistive device to prevent her from falling if she loses her balance. When Alice sees her doctor again in a few months, she should have the bone density test repeated to see if there has been any improvement in bone mass.

At this time, Alice needs to focus first on becoming active again. She will need to eat more food to get enough calories to regain her strength. Also, she needs to add about 700 milligrams of calcium to her daily intake in the form of a calcium carbonate or calcium citrate supplement. An antiresorptive agent should also be added to her medications—either estrogen, a bisphosphonate, or calcitonin. Whichever agent she chooses must be taken consistently because these medications prevent future fractures by almost 50 percent.

Alice's physician should have other recommendations. He should advise her to get information about a local low-impact aerobics class geared to elderly persons with hip fractures and problems related to osteoporosis. Most YMCAs have these classes, as do community centers and local community hospitals. The exercise class will help Alice gain strength and improve her balance, and these improvements will prevent falls. Alice may also need instruction from a physical therapist on how to do things at home so that she does not find herself off balance and ready to take a spill.

Alice's medications will need to be reviewed to find out if any of them can make her drowsy or dizzy. Drowsiness or loss of alertness can lead to falls. Frequently, elderly individuals are given these medications by their doctors for anxiety, insomnia, or chronic pain. Some medications that may cause drowsiness in the elderly include Valium®, librium, sleeping medications including Restoril®, choral hydrate and Benedryl®, and pain medications including Tylenol®, Percoset®, and demerol. All of these medications can cause prolonged drowsiness in the elderly because drugs take much longer to be cleared from the body in older adults, and since many of these persons have chronic ailments, they may take several medications a day. A careful review of all of Alice's medications is very important to prevent another hip fracture.

Appendix: Sources for Further Research

FOUNDATIONS

National Osteoporosis Foundation
1150 17th Street NW
Suite 500
Washington, DC 20036

American Association of Retired Persons
601 E Street NW
Washington, DC 20049

Arthritis Foundation
National Office
1330 West Peachtree Street
Atlanta, GA 30309

National Dairy Council
6300 North River Road
Rosemont, IL 60018-8433

National Institutes of Health
Bethesda, MD 20892

BOOKS ON HEALTH, MENOPAUSE, AND OSTEOPOROSIS
(available in libraries or through the publisher)

Calcium and Common Sense
Robert Heaney, M.D., and M. Janet Barger-Lux, M.S. (1988)

Menopausal Years: The Wise Woman Way
Susan S. Weed
Woodstock, NY
Ash Tree Publishing (1992)

Menopause, Naturally: Preparing for the Second Half of Life (Revised)
S. Greenwood, M.D.
Volcano, CA
Volcano Press (1996)

The Osteoporosis Book
Gwen Ellert, R.N., Med
John Wade, M.D.
Vancouver, BC
Trelle Enterprises (1995; new edition in 1998)

NEWSLETTERS

Harvard Women's Health Watch
Women's Health Advocate
Woman's Health Advisor
P.O. Box 420235
Palm Coast, FL
1-800-829-5921

The Osteoporosis Report
National Osteoporosis Foundation
1150 17th Street NW
Suite 500
Washington, DC 20036

COOKBOOKS

Bone Builders: The Complete Lowfat Cookbook Plus Calcium Health Guide
Edita M. Kaye
New York, NY
Warner Books (1996)

Estrogen: The Natural Way: Delicious Recipes for Menopause
Nina Shandler
New York, NY
Villard Books, A Division of Random House (1997)

Nutrition for Women: The Complete Guide
Elizabeth Somer, M.A., R.D.
New York, NY
Henry Holt & Co. (1994)

The Essential Arthritis Cookbook: Kitchen Basics for People with Arthritis, Fibromyalgia and Other Chronic Pain and Fatigue
Arthritis Center and Department of Nutritional Sciences
University of Alabama at Birmingham
Mankato, MN
Appletree Press (1995)

Bibliography

Introduction

Consensus Development Conference. Diagnosis, prophylaxis and treatment of osteoporosis. *American Journal of Medicine* 94:646–650, 1993.

Cooper, C., Campion, G., and Melton, L. J. Hip fractures in the elderly: A worldwide projection. *Osteoporosis International* 2:285–289, 1992.

Keene, G. S., Parker, J. M., and Pryor, G. A. Mortality and morbidity after hip fractures. *British Medical Journal* 307:1248–1250, 1993.

Melton, J. K., Chrischilles, E. A., Cooper, C., et al. How many women have osteoporosis? *Journal of Bone and Mineral Research* 7:1005–1010, 1992.

Chapter 1

Dempster, D. Bone Remodeling. In Riggs, B. L., and Melton, L. J., III (eds.): *Osteoporosis: Etiology, Diagnosis, and Management,* 2nd ed. Philadelphia: Lippincott-Raven, 1988, pp. 67–91.

Frost, H. M. Dynamics of bone remodeling. In Frost, H. M. (ed.): *Bone Biodynamics.* Boston: Little, Brown, 1964, pp. 315–333.

Hahn, T. J. Steroid and drug-induced osteoporosis. In Favus, M. (ed.): *Primer of Metabolic Bone Diseases and Disorders of Mineral Metabolism.* Philadelphia: Raven, 1997, p. 250.

Mazess, R. B. On aging bone loss. *Clinical Orthopaedics and Related Research* 165:239, 1982.

Riggs, B. L., and Melton, L. J., III. Clinical spectrum. In Riggs, B. L., and Melton, L. J., III. (eds.): *Osteoporosis: Etiology, Diagnosis and Management,* 2nd ed. Philadelphia: Lippincott-Raven, 1988, p. 155.

Stewart, A. F., and Broadus, A. E. Mineral metabolism. In Felig, P., Baxter, J. D., Broadus, A. E., et al. (eds.): *Endocrinology and metabolism,* 2nd ed. New York: McGraw-Hill, pp. 1317–1353, 1987.

Chapter 2

Barzel, U. S. The skeleton as an anion exchange system: Implications for the role of acid-base imbalance and genesis of osteoporosis. *Journal of Bone and Mineral Research* 10:1431–1436, 1995.

Bauer, D. C., Browner, W. S., Cauley, J. A., et al. Factors associated with appendicular bone mass in older women. *Annals of Internal Medicine* 118: 657–665, 1993.

Bickle, D., Cummings, S. R., Genant, G. K., et al. Bone disease in alcohol abuse. *Annals of Internal Medicine* 103:42–48, 1989.

Chapuy, M. C., Arlot, M. E., Duboeuf, F., et al. Vitamin D_3 and calcium to prevent hip fractures in elderly women. *New England Journal of Medicine* 327:1637–1642, 1992.

Chiu, J. F., Lan, S. J., Yang, C. Y., et al. Long-term vegetarian diet and bone mineral density in postmenopausal Taiwanese women. *Calcified Tissue International* 60(3):245–249, 1997.

Cummings, S. R., Black, D. M., and Nevitt, M. C. Bone density at various sites and prediction of hip fracture in women. *Lancet* 341:72–75, 1993.

Cummings, S. R., Kelsey, J. L., and Nevitt, M. C. Epidemiology of osteoporosis and osteoporotic fractures. *Epidemiology Reviews* 7:178–208, 1985.

Ettinger, B. Thyroid supplements: Effects on bone mass. *Western Journal of Medicine* 136:473, 1982.

Hahn, T. J. Steroid and drug-induced osteoporosis. In Favus, M. (ed.): *Primer of Metabolic Bone Diseases and Disorders of Mineral Metabolism.* Philadelphia: Raven Press, 1997, p. 250.

Heaney, R. P., and Recker, R. R. Effects of nitrogen, phosphorus and caffeine on calcium balance in women. *Journal of Laboratory and Clinical Medicine* 99:46–55, 1982.

Johnston, C. C., Peanock, M., and Meunier, P. J. Osteomalacia as a risk factor for hip fractures in the USA. In Christiansen, C., Johansen, J. S., and Riis, B. J. (eds.): *Osteoporosis 1987.* Copenhagen: Osteopress ApS, 1987, pp. 317–320.

Kanis, J. Calcium requirements for optimal skeletal health. *Calcified Tissue International* 49(supplement):S33–S41, 1991.

Lukert, B. P., and Raisz, L. G. Glucocorticoid-induced osteoporosis: Pathogenesis and management. *Annals of Internal Medicine* 1:352–364, 1990.

Marsh, A. G., Sanchez, T. V., Mickelsen, O., et al. Cortical bone density of adult lacto-ovo-vegetarian and omnivorous women. *Journal of the American Dietetic Association* 76:148–151, 1980.

National Institutes of Health (NIH) Consensus Development Panel on Optimal Calcium Intake. Optimal calcium intake. *Journal of the American Medical Association,* 272:1942–1948, 1994.

Nevitt, M. C. Epidemiology of osteoporosis. In Lane, N. E. (ed.): *Osteoporosis. Rheumatic Disease Clinics of North America.* Philadelphia: W. B. Saunders, 1994, pp. 535–560.

Paganini-Hill, A., Chao, A., Ross, R. K., et al. Exercise and other factors in the prevention of hip fractures: The Leisure World Study. *Epidemiology* 2: 16–25, 1991.

Spencer, H., and Lender, M. Adverse effects of aluminum-containing antacids on mineral metabolism. *Gastroenterology* 76:603, 1979.

Wasnich, R., Davis, J., Ross, P., et al. Effects of thiazides on rates of bone loss: A longitudinal study. *British Medical Journal* 301:1303–1305, 1990.

Zhang, J. P., Feldblum, J., and Fortney, S. A. Moderate physical activity and bone density among perimenopausal women. *American Journal of Public Health* 82:736–738, 1992.

Chapter 3

Cummings, S. R., Black, D. M., Nevitt, M. C., et al. Appendicular bone density and age predict hip fracture in women. *Journal of the American Medical Association* 263:665–668, 1990.

Garnero, P., and Delmas, P. D. New developments in biochemical markers of osteoporosis. *Calcified Tissue International* 59:S2–S9, 1996.

Hansen, M., Overgaard, K., Riis, B. J., and Christiansen, C. Role of peak bone mass and bone loss in postmenopausal osteoporosis: 12 year study. *British Medical Journal* 303:961–964, 1991.

Kanis, J. Assessment of bone mass and osteoporosis. In Kanis, J. (ed.): *Osteoporosis.* Oxford: Blackwell Science, 1994, pp. 114–147.

Kanis, J., Melton, L. J., Christiansen, C., et al. The diagnosis of osteoporosis. *Journal of Bone and Mineral Research* 9:1137–1141, 1994.

Kleerekoper, M., and Edelson, G. W. Biochemical studies in the evaluation and management of osteoporosis: Current status and future prospects. *Endocrinology Practice* 2:13–19, 1996.

Lane, N. E., Jergus, M., and Genant, H. K. Osteoporosis and bone mineral density assessment. In Koopman, W. (ed.): *Arthritis and Allied Diseases: A Textbook of Rheumatology*, 13th ed. Baltimore: Williams & Wilkins, 1996, pp. 153–171.

World Health Organization (WHO) Study Group. Assessment of fracture risk and its application to screening for postmenopausal osteoporosis. *WHO Technical Report Series 843.* Geneva: WHO, 1994.

Chapter 4

Barrett-Connor, E. The economic and human costs of osteoporotic fracture. *American Journal of Medicine* 98(Supplement 2A):2A3S–2A8S, 1995.

Cummings, S. R., and Nevitt, M. C. Epidemiology of hip fractures and falls. In Kleerekoper, M., and Krane, S. M. (eds.): *Clinical Disorders of Bone and Mineral Metabolism*. New York: Mary Ann Liebert, Inc., 1989, pp. 231–236.

Cummings, S. R., Nevitt, M. C., Browner, W. S., et al. Risk factors for hip fractures in elderly white women. *New England Journal of Medicine* 332:767–773, 1995.

Eiskjaer, S., Ostgard, S. E., Jakobsen, B. W., et al. Years of potential life lost after hip fracture among postmenopausal women. *Acta Orthopaedic Scandinavica*, 63:293–296, 1992.

Genant, H. K., Wu, C. Y., Van Kauijk, C., et al. Vertebral fracture assessment using a semi-quantitative technique. *Journal of Bone and Mineral Research* 9:1137–1147, 1993.

Kanis, J. Assessment of bone mass and osteoporosis. In Kanis, J. (ed.): *Osteoporosis*. Oxford: Blackwell Science, 1994, pp. 114–147.

Kanis, J. A., and McCloskey, E. V. The epidemiology of vertebral osteoporosis. *Bone* 13 (Supplement 2):S1–S10, 1992.

Keene, G. S., Parker, M. J., and Pryon, G. A. Mortality and morbidity after hip fractures. *British Medical Journal* 307:1248–1250, 1993.

Lips, P., and Obrant, K. J. The pathogenesis and treatment of hip fractures. *Osteoporosis International* 1:218–231, 1991.

Melton, L. J., III, Kan, S. H., Frye, M. A., et al. Epidemiology of vertebral fractures in women. *American Journal of Epidemiology* 129:1000–1011, 1989.

Melton, L. J., III, and Riggs, B. L. Risk factors for injury after a fall. *Clinics in Geriatric Medicine* 1:525–539, 1985.

Nevitt, M. C., and Cummings, S. R. Falls and fractures in older women. In Vellas, B., Troupet, M., Rubenstein, L., et al. (eds.): *Falls, Balance and Gait: Disorders in the Elderly*. Paris: Elsevier, 1992, pp. 69–80.

Nevitt, M. C., and Cummings, S. R. Type of fall and risk of hip and wrist fractures: The study of osteoporotic fractures. *Journal of the American Geriatric Society* 41:1226–1234.

White, B. L., Fisher, W. D., and Laurin, C. A. Rate of mortality for elderly patients after fracture of the hip in the 1980s. *Journal of Bone and Joint Surgery* 69A:1335–1339, 1987.

Chapter 5

Allain, T., Pitt, P., and Moniz, C. Osteoporosis in men. *British Medical Journal*, 305:955–956, 1992.

Jackson, J. A. Osteoporosis in men. In Flavus, M. (ed.): *Primer of Metabolic Bone Diseases and Disorders of Mineral Metabolism*, 2nd ed. Philadelphia: Raven Press, 1993, pp. 255–258.

Jackson, J. A., and Kleerekoper, M. Osteoporosis in men: Diagnosis, pathophysiology and prevention. *Medicine* 69:139–152, 1990.

Orwoll, E. S., and Klein, R. F. Osteoporosis in men. *Endocrine Reviews* 16:87–116, 1995.

Seaman, E., and Melton, L. J., III Risk factor for spinal osteoporosis in men. *American Journal of Medicine* 75:977–983, 1983.

Chapter 6

Bush, T. L., Barrett-Connor, E., Cowan, L. D., et al. Cardiovascular mortality and noncontraceptive use of estrogen in women: Results from the Lipid Research Clinics Program Follow-up study. *Circulation* 75:112–119, 1987.

Cauley, J., Seeley, D. G., Ensrud, K., et al. Estrogen replacement and fracture protection in older women. *Annals of Internal Medicine* 122:9–16, 1995.

Colditz, G. A., Hankinson, S. E., Hunter, D. J., et al. The use of estrogens and progestins and the risk of breast cancer in postmenopausal women. *New England Journal of Medicine* 332:1589–1593, 1995.

Grady, D., Rubin, S. M., Petitti, D., et al. Hormone therapy to prevent disease and prolong life in postmenopausal women. *Annals of Internal Medicine* 117:1016–1037, 1992.

Greenwood, S. All about hot flashes and how to live with them. In Greenwood, S.: *Menopause, Naturally* (updated). Volcano, CA: Volcano Press, 1992, pp. 29–40.

Ingram, D., Sander, K., Kolybaba, M., et al. Case-control study of phytoestrogens and breast cancer. *Lancet* 350(9083):990–994, 1997.

Kiel, D. P., Felson, D. T., Anderson, J. J., et al. Hip fracture and the use of estrogen in postmenopausal women. The Framingham Study. *New England Journal of Medicine* 317:1169–1174, 1987.

Knight, D. C., and Eden, J. A. A review of the clinical effects of phytoestrogens. *Obstetrics and Gynecology* 87:897–904, 1996.

Lien, L. L., and Lien, E. J. Hormone therapy and phytoestrogens. *Journal of Clinical Pharmacy and Therapeutics* 21(2):101–111, 1996.

Lindsay, R. Prevention and treatment of osteoporosis. *Lancet* 341:801–805, 1993.

Lindsay, R., Aitken, J. M., Anderson, J. B., et al. Long-term prevention of post-menopausal osteoporosis by estrogen. *Lancet* 1:1038–1041, 1976.

Lindsay, R., and Tohme, J. F. Estrogen treatment of patients with established postmenopausal osteoporosis. *Obstetrics and Gynecology* 76:290–295, 1990.

Love, R. R., Barden, H. S., Mazess, R. B., et al. Effect of tamoxifen on lumbar spine bone mineral density in postmenopausal women after 5 years. *Archives of Internal Medicine* 154:2585–2588, 1994.

Lufkin, E. G., Wahner, H. W., O'Fallon, W. M., et al. Treatment of postmenopausal osteoporosis with transdermal estrogen. *Annals of Internal Medicine* 117:1–9, 1992.

Lukfin, E. G., Whitaker, M. D., Argueta, R., et al. Raloxifene treatment of postmenopausal osteoporosis. *Journal of Bone and Mineral Research* 12(Supplement 1):S150, 1997.

Paganini-Hill, A., and Henderson, V. W. Estrogen deficiency and risk of Alzheimer's disease in women. *American Journal of Epidemiology* 140:256–261, 1994.

Physicians Desk Reference, 51st ed. Montvale, NJ: Medical Economics, 1997.

Ryan, P. J., Harrison, R., Blake, G. M., et al. Compliance with hormone replacement therapy (HRT) after screening for postmenopausal osteoporosis. *British Journal of Obstetrics and Gynecology* 99:325–328, 1992.

Stanford, J. L., Weiss, N. S., Voigt, L. F., et al. The use of estrogens and progestins and the risk of breast cancer in postmenopausal women. *Journal of the American Medical Association* 274:137–142, 1995.

Taylor, M. Alternatives to conventional hormone replacement therapy. *Comprehensive Therapy* 23(8):514–532, 1997.

Chapter 7

Aloia, J. F., Vaswani, A., Yeh, J. K., et al. Calcium supplementation with and without hormone replacement therapy to prevent postmenopausal bone loss. *Annals of Internal Medicine* 120:97–103, 1994.

Dawson-Hughes, D., Dallal, G. E., Krall, E. A., et al. A controlled trial of the effect of calcium supplementation on bone density in postmenopausal women. *New England Journal of Medicine* 328:460, 1993.

Elders, P. J. M., Netelenbos, J. C., Lips, P., et al. Calcium supplementation reduces vertebral bone loss in perimenopausal women: A controlled trial in 248 women between 46 and 55 years of age. *Journal of Clinical Endocrinology and Metabolism* 73:533–540, 1991.

Heaney, R. P. Thinking straight about calcium. *New England Journal of Medicine* 328:503, 1993.

Johnson, C. C., Jr., Miller, J. Z., Slemenda, C. W., et al. Calcium supplementation and increases in bone mineral density in children. *New England Journal of Medicine* 327:82–87, 1992.

National Institutes of Health (NIH) Consensus Development Panel on Optimal Calcium Intake. Optimal calcium intake. *Journal of the American Medical Association* 272:1942–1948, 1994.

Recker, R. R., Davies, K. M., Hinders, S. M., et al. Bone gain in young adult women. *Journal of the American Medical Association* 268:2403–2408, 1992.

Recker, R. R., Hinders, S., Davies, K. M., et al. Correcting calcium nutritional deficiency prevents spine fractures in elderly women. *Journal of Bone Mineral Research* 11:1961–1966, 1996.

Reid, I. R., Ames, R. W., Evans, M. C., et al. Effect of calcium supplementation on bone loss in postmenopausal women. *New England Journal of Medicine* 323:878–881, 1990.

Bisphosphonates

Black, D. M., Cummings, S. R., Karpt, D. B., et al. Randomised trial of effect of alendronate on risk of fracture in women with existing vertebral fractures. *Lancet* 348:1535–1541, 1996.

Fleisch, H. Bisphosphonates. *Drugs* 42:919–944, 1991.

Harris, S. T., Watts, N. B., Jackson, R. D., et al. Four year study of intermittent cyclic etidronate treatment of postmenopausal osteoporosis: Three years of blinded therapy. *American Journal of Medicine* 95:285, 1992.

Liberman, U. A., Weiss, S. R., Broll, J., et al: Effect of alendronate on bone mineral density and the incidence of fracture in postmenopausal osteoporotic women. *New England Journal of Medicine* 1:1130–1131, 1995.

Rodan, G. A., and Fleisch, H. A. Bisphosphonates: Mechanism of action. *Journal of Clinical Investigation* 97:2692–2696, 1996.

Storm, T., Thamsborg, G., Steiniche, T., et al. Effect of intermittent cyclical etidronate therapy on bone mass and fracture rate in women with postmenopausal osteoporosis. *New England Journal of Medicine* 322:1265, 1990.

Watts, N. Treatment of osteoporosis with bisphosphonates. In Lane, N. E. (ed.): *Osteoporosis. Rheumatic Disease Clinics of North America.* Philadelphia: W. B. Saunders, 1994, pp. 717–734.

Watts, N. B., Harris, S. T., Genant, H. K., et al. Intermittent cyclical etidronate treatment of postmenopausal osteoporosis. *New England Journal of Medicine* 323:73–79, 1990.

Calcitonin

Avioli, L. V. Calcitonin therapy for osteoporotic syndromes. In Lane, N. E. (ed.): *Osteoporosis. Rheumatic Disease Clinics of North America*. Philadelphia: W. B. Saunders, 1994, pp. 777–786.

Civitelli, R., Gonnelli, S., Zacchei, F., et al. Bone turnover in postmenopausal osteoporosis: Effect of calcitonin treatment. *Journal of Clinical Investigation* 82:1268–1274, 1988.

Lyritis, G. P., Tsakalabos, S., Magiasis, B., et al. Analgesic effect of salmon calcitonin on osteoporotic vertebral fractures. Double-blind, placebo-controlled study. *Calcified Tissue International* 49:369–372, 1982.

Overgaard, K. Y., Hansen, M. A., Jensen, J. B., et al. Effect of salcatonin given intranasally on bone mass and fracture rates in established osteoporosis: A dose-response study. *British Medical Journal* 305:556–561, 1992.

Overgaard, K., Riis, B. J., Christiansen, C., et al. Effect of salcatonin given intranasally on early postmenopausal bone loss. *British Journal of Medicine* 299:477–479, 1989.

Reginster, J. Y. Effect of calcitonin on bone mass and fracture rates. *American Journal of Medicine* 91 (Supplement 5B):19–22, 1991.

Chapter 8

Bickle, D. D. Role of vitamin D, its metabolites, and analogs in the management of osteoporosis. In Lane, N. E. (ed.): *Osteoporosis. Rheumatic Disease Clinics of North America*. Philadelphia: W. B. Saunders, 1994, pp. 759–775.

Bullamore, J. R., Gallagher, J. C., Wilkinson, R., et al. Effect of age on calcium absorption. *Lancet* 1:535–537, 1977.

Chapuy, M. C., Arlot, M. E., Duboeuf, F., et al. Vitamin D_3 and calcium prevent hip fractures in elderly women. *New England Journal of Medicine* 327:1637–1642, 1992.

Dawson-Hughes, B., Dallal, G. E., Krall, E. A., et al. Effect of vitamin D supplementation on wintertime and overall bone loss in healthy postmenopausal women. *Annals of Internal Medicine* 115:502–512, 1991.

Gallagher, J. C., Beneton, M., Harvey. L, et al. Response of rachitic rat bones to 1,25-dihydroxyvitamin D_3: Biphasic effects on mineralization and lack of effect on bone resorption. *Endocrinology* 119:1603–1609, 1986.

Gallagher, J. C., Riggs, B. L., Eisman, J., et al. Intestinal calcium absorption and serum vitamin D metabolites in normal subjects and osteoporotic subjects: Effect of age and dietary calcium. *Journal of Clinical Investigation* 64:613–617, 1979.

Gennari, C., Agnudei, D., Nardi, P., et al. Estrogen preserves a normal intestinal responsiveness to 1,25-dihydroxyvitamin D_3 in oophorectomized women. *Journal of Clinical Endocrinology and Metabolism* 71:1288–1293, 1990.

Glorieux, F. H. Calcitriol treatment in vitamin D-dependent and vitamin D-resistant rickets. *Metabolism* 39 (Supplement 1):10–12, 1990.

Sowers, M. R. Epidemiology of calcium and vitamin D in bone loss. *Journal of Nutrition* 123:413–417, 1993.

Tilyard, M. W., Spears, G. F. S., Thomson, J., et al. Treatment of postmenopausal osteoporosis with calcitriol and calcium. *New England Journal of Medicine* 326:357–362, 1992.

Vitamin D Receptor and Bone Mass

Riggs, B. L., Nguyen, T. V., Melton, J. L., III, et al. The contribution of vitamin D receptor gene alleles to the determination of bone mineral density in normal and osteoporotic women. *Journal of Bone and Mineral Research* 10:991–996, 1995.

Vandevyver, C., Wylin, T., Cassiman, J. J., et al. Influence of the vitamin D receptor alleles on bone mineral density in postmenopausal and osteoporotic women. *Journal of Bone and Mineral Research* 12:241–247, 1997.

Chapter 9

Barrow, G. W., and Saha, S. Menstrual irregularity and stress fractures in collegiate female distance runners. *Journal of American Sports Medicine* 16:209–216, 1988.

Bouxsein, M. L., and Marcus R. Overview of exercise and bone mass. In Lane, N. E. (ed): *Osteoporosis. Rheumatic Disease Clinics of North America.* Philadelphia: W. B. Saunders, 1994, pp. 787–802.

Chow, R., Harrison, J. E., and Dornan, J. Prevention and rehabilitation of osteoporosis: Exercise and osteoporosis. *International Journal of Rehabilitation Research* 12:49–56, 1989.

Chow, R., Harrison, J. E., and Notarius, C. Effect of two randomised exercise programmes on bone mass of healthy postmenopausal women. *British Journal of Medicine* 295:1441–1444, 1987.

Constantini, N. W., and Warren, M. P. Special problems in the female athlete. In Panush, R. S., and Lane, N. E. (eds.): *Bailliere's Clinical Rheumatology—Exercise and Rheumatic Disease*, Vol. 8, No. 10. London: Ballière Tindall, 1994, pp. 199–219.

Dale, E., Gerlach, D. H., and Wilhite, A. L. Menstrual dysfunction in distance runners. *Obstetrics and Gynecology* 54:47–53, 1979.

Dalen, N., and Olsson, K. E. Bone mineral content and physical activity. *Acta Orthopaedic Scandinavica* 45:170–174, 1974.

Dalsky, G. P., Stocke, K. S., Ehsani, A. A., et al. Weight-bearing exercise training and lumbar bone mineral content in postmenopausal women. *Annals of Internal Medicine* 108:824–828, 1988.

Douglas, P. S., Clarkson, T. B., Flowers, N. C., et al. Exercise and atherosclerotic heart disease in women. *Medicine and Science in Sports and Exercise* 24:266–276, 1992.

Drinkwater, B. L., Nilson, K., Chestnut, C. H., et al. Bone mineral content of amenorrheic and eumenorrheic athletes. *New England Journal of Medicine* 311:277–281, 1984.

Drinkwater, B. L., Nilson, K., Ott, S., et al. Bone mineral density after resumption of menses in amenorrheic athletes. *Journal of the American Medical Association* 256:380–382, 1986.

Frisch, R. E., Gotz-Welbergen, A. V., McArthur, J. W., et al. Delayed menarche and amenorrhea of college athletes in relation to age of onset of training. *Journal of the American Medical Association* 246:1559–1563, 1981.

Krolner, B., Toft, B., Nielsen, S. P., et al. Physical exercise as prophylaxis against involutional vertebral bone loss: A controlled trial. *Clinical Science* 64:541–546, 1983.

Lamon-Fava, S., Fisher, E. C., Nelson, M. E., et al. Effect of exercise and menstrual cycle status on plasma lipids, low density lipoprotein particle size, and apolipoproteins. *Journal of Clinical Endocrinology and Metabolism* 68:17–21, 1989.

Lane, N. E., Bloch, D., Jones, H. H., et al. Long-distance running, bone density and osteoarthritis. *Journal of the American Medical Association* 255: 1147–1151, 1986.

Lane, N. E., Bloch, D., Jones, H. H., et al. Running, osteoarthritis, and bone density: Initial longitudinal study. *American Journal of Medicine* 88: 452–459, 1989.

Leicheter, I., Simkin, A., Margulies, J. Y., et al. Gain in mass density of bone following strenuous physical activity. *Journal of Orthopaedic Research* 7:86–90, 1984.

Michel, B. A., Lane, N. E., Bjorkenaren, A., et al. Impact of running on lumbar bone density: A 5-year longitudinal study. *Journal of Rheumatology* 19: 1759–1763, 1992.

Nelson, M. E., Meredith, C. N., Dawson-Hughes, B., et al. Hormone and bone mineral status in endurance-trained and sedentary postmenopausal women. *Journal of Clinical Endocrinology and Metabolism* 66:927–933, 1988.

Notelovitz, M., Martin, D., Tesar, R., et al. Estrogen therapy and variable-resistance weight-training increase bone mineral in surgically menopausal women. *Journal of Bone and Mineral Research* 6:583–590, 1991.

Prince, R. L., Smith, M., and Dick, I. M. Prevention of postmenopausal osteoporosis: A comparative study of exercise, calcium supplementation, and hormone-replacement therapy. *New England Journal of Medicine* 325: 1189–1195, 1991.

Pruitt, L., Jackson, R., Bartels, R., et al. Weight-training effects on bone mineral density in early postmenopausal women. *Journal of Bone and Mineral Research* 7:179–185, 1992.

Recker, R. R., Davies, K. M., Hinders, S. M., et al. Bone gain in young adult women. *Journal of the American Medical Association* 268:2403–2408, 1992.

Rosen, L. W., McKeag, D. B., Hough, D. O., et al. Pathogenic weight-control behavior in female athletes. *The Physician and Sportsmedicine* 14:79–86, 1986.

Sinaki, M., and Mikkelsen, B. Postmenopausal spinal osteoporosis: Flexion versus extension exercises. *Archives of Physical Medicine and Rehabilitation* 65:593–596, 1984.

Snead, D. B., Stubbs, C. C., Weltman, J. Y., et al. Dietary patterns, eating behaviors, and bone mineral density in women runners. *American Journal of Clinical Nutrition* 56:705–711, 1992.

Warren, M. P. The effects of exercise on pubertal progression and reproductive function in girls. *Journal of Clinical Endocrinology and Metabolism* 51: 1150–1157, 1980.

Warren, M. P., Brooks-Gunn, J., Fox, R. P., et al. Scoliosis and fractures in young ballet dancers: Relation to delayed menarche and secondary amenorrhea. *New England Journal of Medicine* 314:1348–1353, 1986.

Welten, D. C., et al. Weight-bearing activity during youth is a more important factor for peak bone mass than calcium intake. *Journal of Bone and Mineral Research* 9:1089–1096, 1994.

Chapter 10

Finkelstein, J. S., Klibanski, A., Schaefer, E. H., et al. Parathyroid hormone for the prevention of bone loss induced by estrogen deficiency. *New England Journal of Medicine* 331: 1618–1623, 1994.

Kimmel, D. B., Slovik, D. M., and Lane, N. E. Current and investigational approaches for reversing established osteoporosis. In Lane, N. E. (ed.), *Osteoporosis. Rheumatic Disease Clinics of North America.* Philadelphia: W. B. Saunders, 1994, pp. 735–758.

Kleerekoper, M., and Medlovic, D. B. Sodium fluoride therapy of postmenopausal osteoporosis. *Endocrine Reviews* 14:312–323, 1993.

Lindsay, R., Nieves, J., Formica, C., et al. Randomized controlled clinical trial of the effect of parathyroid hormone on vertebral bone mass and fracture incidence among postmenopausal women on estrogen with osteoporosis. *Lancet* 350:550–556, 1997.

Neer, R. M., Slovik, D., Doppelt, S., et al. The use of parathyroid hormone plus 1,25(OH)2D3 to increase trabecular bone in osteoporotic men and post-menopausal women. In Christiansen, C., Johansen, J. S., and Riis, B. J. (eds.): *Osteoporosis 1987.* Copenhagen: Osteopress ApS, 1987, pp. 829–835.

Pak, C. Y., Saghaeek, K., Adams-Huet, B., et al. Treatment of postmenopausal osteoporosis with slow-release sodium fluoride. Final report of a randomized controlled trial. *Annals of Internal Medicine* 123:40–1408, 1995.

Riggs, B. L., Hodgson, S. F., O'Fallon, W. M., et al. Effect of fluoride treatment on the fracture rate in postmenopausal women with osteoporosis. *New England Journal of Medicine* 322:802–809, 1990.

Chapter 11

Adachi, J. D., Bensen, W. G., Bianchi, F., et al. Vitamin D and calcium in the prevention of corticosteroid induced osteoporosis: A 3 year follow-up study. *Journal of Rheumatology* 23:995–1000, 1996.

Adachi, J. D., Benson, W. G., Brown, J., et al. Etidronate therapy to prevent corticosteroid-induced osteoporosis. *New England Journal of Medicine* 337(6): 382–387, 1997.

Adler, R. A., and Rosen, C. J. Glucocorticoids and osteoporosis. *Endocrinology and Metabolism Clincs of North America* 23: 641–654, 1994.

Buckley, L., Leib, E., Cartularo, K. S., et al. Calcium and Vitamin D_3 supplementation prevents bone loss in the spine secondary to low dose corticosteroids in patients with rheumatoid arthritis. *Annals of Internal Medicine* 125:961–968, 1996.

Hall, G. M., Daniels, M., Doyle, D. V., et al. Effect of hormone replacement therapy on bone mass in rheumatoid arthritis patients treated with and without steroids. *Arthritis and Rheumatism* 37:1499–1505, 1994.

Luengo, M., Picado, C., Del Rio, L., et al. Treatment of steroid-induced ostopenia with calcitonin in corticosteroid-dependent asthma: A one-year follow-up study. *American Review of Respiratory Disease* 142:104–107, 1990.

Lukert, B. P., Johnson, B. E., and Robinson, R. G. Estrogen and progesterone replacement therapy reduces glucocorticoid induced bone loss. *Journal of Bone and Mineral Research* 7:1063–1069, 1992.

Lukert, B. P., and Raisz, L. G. Glucocorticoid-induced osteoporosis. In Lane, N. E. (ed.): *Osteoporosis. Rheumatic Disease Clinics of North America.* Philadelphia: W. B. Saunders, 1994, pp. 629–650.

Reid, I. R., King, A. R., Alexander, C. J., et al. Prevention of steroid-induced osteoporosis with (3-amino-1-hydroxypropylidene) 1,1-bisphosphonate (APD). *Lancet* 1:143–146, 1988.

Reid, I. R., Wattie, D. J., Evans, M. C., et al. Testosterone therapy in glucocorticoid-treated men. *Archives of Internal Medicine* 156:1173–1177, 1996.

Ringe, J. D. Intranasal salmon calcitonin in the treatment of steroid-induced osteoporosis. In Christiansen, C., and Overgaard, K. (eds.): *Osteoporosis 1990.* Copenhagen: Osteopress ApS, 1990, pp. 1868–1871.

Sambrook, P. N., Birmingham, J., Kelly, P., et al. Prevention of corticosteroid osteoporosis. A comparison of calcium, calcitriol and calcitonin. *New England Journal of Medicine* 328:1747–1752, 1993.

Chapter 12

Gold, D. T., and Drezner, M. K. Quality of life. In Riggs, B. L., and Melton, L. J., III (eds.): *Osteoporosis: Etiology, Diagnosis, and Management,* 2nd ed. Philadelphia: Lipppincott-Raven, 1995, pp. 475–486

Gold, D. T., Lyles, K. W., Blaes, C. W., et al. Teaching patients coping behaviors: An essential part of successful management of osteoporosis. *Journal of Bone and Mineral Research* 4:799–801, 1989.

Itoi, E., and Sanaki, M. Effect of back-strengthening exercise on posture in healthy women 49 to 65 years of age. *Mayo Clinic Proceedings* 69:1054–1059, 1994.

Kaplan, R. S., Sinaki, M., and Hameister, M. D. Effect of back supports on back strength in patients with osteoporosis: A pilot study. *Mayo Clinic Proceedings* 71:235–241, 1996.

Knapp, M. E. Massage. In Kottke, F. J., and Lehmann, J. F. (eds.): *Krusen's Handbook of Physical Medicine and Rehabilitation,* 4th ed. Philadelphia: W. B. Saunders, 1990, pp. 433–435.

Lehmann, J. F., and DeLateur, B. J. Diathermy and superficial heat, laser and cold therapy. In Kottke, F. J., and Lehmann, J. F. (eds.): *Krusen's Handbook of Physical Medicine and Rehabilitation,* 4th ed. Philadelphia: W. B. Saunders, 1990, pp. 283–367.

National Osteoporosis Foundation Handbook on Exercises for Women with Osteoporosis. Washington, DC: National Osteoporosis Foundation.

Sinaki, M. Musculoskeletal rehabilitation. In Riggs, B. L., and Melton, J. L., III (eds.): *Osteoporosis: Etiology, Diagnosis, and Management*, 2nd ed. Philadelphia: Lippincott-Raven, 1995, pp. 435–471.

Sinaki, M. Postmenopausal spinal osteoporosis: Physical therapy and rehabilitative principles. *Mayo Clinic Proceedings* 57:699–675, 1992.

Sinaki, M., Dale., D. A., and Hurley, D. L. *Living with Osteoporosis: Guidelines for Women Before and After Diagnosis.* Toronto: B. C. Decker, 1988.

Sinaki, M., Itoi, E., Rogers, J. W., et al. Correlation of back extensor strength with thoracic kyphosis and lumbar lordosis in estrogen-deficient women. *American Journal of Physical Medicine and Rehabilitation* 75:370–374, 1996.

Urist, M. R. Orthopaedic management of osteoporosis in postmenopausal women. *Clinical Endocrinology and Metabolism* 2:159–176, 1973.

Index